EMQs

for surgery

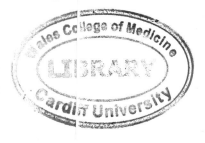

Edited by Louis J Fligelstone & Alun H Davies

tfm Publishing Ltd, Castle Hill Barns, Harley, Nr Shrewsbury, SY5 6LX, UK.
Tel: +44 (0)1952 510061; Fax: +44 (0)1952 510192
E-mail: nikki@tfmpublishing.com; Web site: www.tfmpublishing.com

Design and layout: Nikki Bramhill

Copyright © 2005 tfm publishing Ltd.

ISBN 1 903378 15 X

Printed by Gutenberg Press Ltd., Gudja Road, Tarxien, PLA 19, Malta.

Tel: +356 21897037; Fax: +356 21800069.

Contents

Contributors

Bilal A Al-Sarireh MRCS (Ed) PhD (Eng), Specialist Registrar, General Surgery, Morriston Hospital, Swansea, UK

Yogesh Bajaj MS MRCS (Ed), Research Fellow, Otolaryngology, Great Ormond Street, London, UK

Aidan Byrne MD MRCP FRCA, Consultant Anaesthetist, Morriston Hospital, Swansea, UK

Mike Chare MA BM BCh FRCS, Consultant Breast & General Surgeon, Morriston Hospital, Swansea, UK

Alun H Davies MA DM FRCS, Reader in Surgery and Consultant Surgeon, Imperial College School of Medicine, Charing Cross Hospital, London, UK

Meryl Davis FRCS, Specialist Registrar, Surgery, Imperial College School of Medicine, Charing Cross Hospital, London, UK

Mriganka De MRCS (Ed) MRCS (Glas), Specialist Registrar, Otolaryngology, West Midlands Rotation, UK

Peter Drew MB BCh (Wales) FRCS (Eng) FRCS (Ed) FRCS (Plast), Consultant in Plastic and Reconstructive Surgery, Morriston Hospital, Swansea, UK

Sean Dwyer MB BS FRCA, Consultant Anaesthetist, Morriston Hospital, Swansea, UK

Neil J Fenn MB BCh FRCS (Ed) FRCS (Urol), Consultant Urologist, Morriston Hospital, Swansea, UK

Louis J Fligelstone MB BCh MD FRCS (Eng) FRCS (Gen), Consultant Surgeon, Morriston Hospital, Swansea, UK

Damien Kelleher FRCS, Staff Grade, Surgery, Morriston Hospital, Swansea, UK

Michele E Lucarotti MD FRCS, Consultant Surgeon, Gloucestershire Royal Hospital, Gloucester, UK

Heyman Luckraz MB BS FRCS, Specialist Registrar, Cardiothoracic Surgery, Morriston Hospital, Swansea, UK

Aileen McKinley FRCS, Consultant Surgeon, Aberdeen Royal Infirmary, Aberdeen, UK

Terry O'Kelly MD FRCS, Consultant Surgeon, Aberdeen Royal Infirmary, Aberdeen, UK

Robert Redfern FRCS, Consultant Neurosurgeon, Morriston Hospital, Swansea, UK

Stuart Roy MB ChB Mphil (Cantab) FRCS (Ed) Tr & Orth, Specialist Registrar, Trauma & Orthopaedics, Morriston Hospital, Swansea, UK

Gareth Tervit FRCS, Consultant Vascular Surgeon, University Hospital of North Durham, Durham, UK

Mark Vipond MS FRCS, Consultant Surgeon, Gloucestershire Royal Hospital, Gloucester, UK

Paul Williams BSc (Hons) MB BCh FRCS (Eng) FRCS Tr & Orth, Consultant Trauma & Orthopaedic Surgeon, Morriston Hospital, Swansea, UK

Afzal Zaidi MA MB BChir FRCS (C-Th), Consultant Cardiothoracic Surgeon, Morriston Hospital, Swansea, UK

Foreword

The assessment of medical knowledge is evolving. Extended Matching Questions (EMQs) are fast becoming one of the preferred structured question assessments of how well medical knowledge is applied in the clinical setting, both in medical schools and for subsequent professional examinations.

The need to practise answering this type of question may often make the difference between passing and failing such an examination. It is hoped that this book will not only help the reader pass examinations, but more importantly, acquire knowledge to support their development into competent and knowledgeable surgeons.

The editors of this book have enlisted the help of specialists in all relevant clinical specialties to create a large bank of questions typical of the assessment of candidates in postgraduate examinations such as the MRCS/FRCS in the United Kingdom. It is likely that the Board Exams in the United States may also follow this question structure.

It is hoped that this book will be an invaluable asset for those preparing for examinations as well as an important part of the self-assessment process at all levels.

When working through the questions it is important to remember that each option may be used once, more than once or not at all. When options appear in brackets within the answers, this indicates a less favoured option.

Louis J Fligelstone & Alun H Davies
Editors
October 2004

Chapter 1

Basic surgical knowledge

Alun H Davies, MA DM FRCS
Reader in Surgery and Consultant Surgeon
Meryl Davis, FRCS
Specialist Registrar, Sugery
Imperial College School of Medicine, Charing Cross Hospital, London, UK
Louis J Fligelstone, MB BCh FRCS (Eng) FRCS (Gen)
Consultant Surgeon, Morriston Hospital, Swansea, UK

For all questions each option may be used once, more than once or not at all.

Question 1. **Wound management and closure techniques**

Match the types of wound to appropriate management.

Options

1   Interrupted nylon suture.
2   Subcuticular absorbable suture.
3   Skin staples.
4   Tissue glue.
5   Steristrips.
6   Delayed primary closure.
7   Heal by second intention.
8   Surgical debridement.
9   Larval therapy.

Stems

A   Superficial wound dehiscence.
B   Perforated appendix.
C   Inflamed appendix.
D   Clean incised superficial skin wound.
E   Grossly contaminated wound.
F   Necrotic, sloughy wound.
G   Non-healing.
H   Granulating.

Question 2. Classification of wounds

Options

1 Elective colorectal resection.
2 Perforated viscus.
3 Perforated appendix.
4 Open cholecystectomy.
5 Excision of skin lesion.
6 Amputation.
7 Laparoscopic cholecystectomy.
8 Open or laparoscopic hernia repair.

Stems

A Clean.
B Clean contaminated.
C Dirty.

Question 3. Anastomoses

Match the technique to the disease.

Options

1 Circular stapling device.
2 3/0 prolene.
3 6/0 prolene.
4 3/0 Monocryl®.
5 3/0 Vicryl Rapide®.
6 GIA stapler.

Stems

A Partial gastrectomy.
B Aortic aneurysm repair.
C Low anterior resection.

D   Carotid endarterectomy.
E   Skin closure forearm.
F   Small bowel anastomosis.
G   Appendicectomy.

Question 4. Aetiology of anastomotic complications

Match the following.

Options

1   Ischaemia.
2   Tension.
3   Stapled anastomosis.
4   Infection.
5   Poor tissue handling.
6   Hand-sewn anastomosis.
7   Distal obstruction.
8   Suture failure.

Stems

A   Stomal prolapse.
B   Anastomotic breakdown.
C   Stomal stenosis.
D   False aneurysm formation.
E   Stoma retraction.

Question 5. Minimally invasive surgery

Match the technique to the pathology.

Options

1   Laparoscopic surgery is standard.
2   Laparoscopic surgery is contraindicated.
3   Laparoscopic treatment is increasingly common.
4   Laparoscopic surgery may have a role in the future.
5   Open surgery is mandatory.
6   Open surgery is currently favoured.
7   Endovascular repair is frequently used.
8   Percutaneous balloon angioplasty.

Stems

A   Aortoiliac occlusive disease.
B   Radical nephrectomy.
C   Cholecystectomy.
D   Common bile duct stone retrieval.
E   Pyeloplasty.
F   Aortic aneurysm repair.
G   Radical cystectomy.
H   Large colonic tumour.

Question 6. Complications of laparoscopy

Match the following.

Options

1   Improved visualisation of tissues and reduced risk of damage to viscera.
2   Never associated with bowel perforation.
3   Gas embolism.
4   Is only used by gynaecologists.
5   Retroperitoneal approach to viscera.
6   Increased risk of injury to bladder, bowel and major blood vessels.

Stems

A   Veress needle.
B   Hassan technique.
C   Insufflation with nitrous oxide.
D   Insufflation pressure of >20mmHg.
E   Balloon dissector.

Question 7. Obstruction

Match the following.

Options

1   Distended abdomen.
2   Bile-stained vomiting.
3   Old food (several meals old).
4   Recently swallowed food without acidic taste.
5   Waterbrash.
6   Nocturnal asthma.
7   Aspiration pneumonitis.
8   Faeculent vomiting.
9   Succussion splash.
10   Vomiting faeces.

Stems

A   Low small bowel obstruction.
B   Gastric outlet obstruction.
C   High small bowel obstruction.
D   Gastrocolic fistula.
E   Achalasia.
F   Oesophageal reflux.
G   Adhesive obstruction.

Question 8. Abdominal wall / hernia

Match the following.

Options

1   Parastomal hernia.
2   Incisional hernia.
3   Inguinal hernia.
4   Femoral hernia.
5   Umbilical hernia.
6   Paraumbilical hernia.
7   Prevascular hernia.
8   Gilmore's groin.
9   Recurrent inguinal hernia.

Stems

A   PHS mesh.
B   Perfix plug.
C   Bassini repair.
D   Laparoscopic hernia repair.
E   Lichtenstein repair.
F   Simple suture.
G   Mayo repair.
H   Mesh repair.
I   Nyhus preperitoneal repair.
J   Permacol (porcine skin).

Question 9. Landmarks for examination of herniae

Options

1   Greater trochanter.
2   Pubic tubercle.
3   Ischial spine.
4   Half way between symphysis pubis and anterior superior iliac spine.

5 Femoral artery.
6 Half way between the anterior superior iliac spine and pubic tubercle.
7 Anterior superior iliac spine.
8 1cm above the midpoint of the inguinal ligament.
9 4cm below and lateral to the pubic tubercle.
10 Half way between the pubic tubercle and the umbilicus.

Stems

A Mid inguinal point.
B Midpoint of the inguinal ligament.
C Landmarks for inguinal ligament.
D Landmark for deep inguinal ring.
E Landmark for the saphenofemoral junction.

Question 10. Identification of viscera

Options

1 Moves down on inspiration.
2 Enlarges in the direction of the right iliac fossa.
3 Enlarges in the direction of the left iliac fossa.
4 Can be balloted.
5 Cannot get between the organ and the costal margin.
6 Mobile.
7 Has a medial notch.
8 Upper and lower limits must be defined to distinguish between displacement and enlargement.
9 Leaning the patient ('tilting') can help identify moderate enlargement.
10 Can get between the organ and the costal margin.
11 Is not palpable until reaching twice its normal size.
12 Dull to percussion.
13 Resonant to percussion.

Stems

A   Cervix.
B   Spleen.
C   Liver.
D   Kidney.
E   Bladder.
F   Ovary.
G   Foetus.

Question 11. Blood products and blood transfusion

Options

1   5% dextrose.
2   Autologous cell salvage.
3   Haemodilution.
4   Pre-operative donation and storage.
5   EPO therapy.
6   Group-specific blood.
7   0 positive blood.
8   Haemoglobin solutions.

Stems

A   Clean abdominal surgery.
B   Joint revision surgery.
C   Cancer surgery.
D   Contaminated abdominal surgery.
E   Abdominal aortic aneurysm surgery.
F   Major cardiac surgery.
G   Elective surgery in high-risk renal patients.
H   Jehovah's witnesses.

Question 12. Classical x-ray signs

Options

1   Lightbulb sign.
2   Double bubble sign.
3   Looser's zones.
4   Boot-shaped heart.
5   Widened mediastinum.
6   Owl's eye sign.
7   Dilated small bowel.
8   Sail sign.
9   Coffee bean sign.
10   Air in biliary tree.
11   Teeth in pelvis.

Stems

A   Tetralogy of Fallot.
B   Posterior dislocation of the shoulder.
C   Thoracic aortic aneurysm.
D   Vertebral fracture.
E   Gallstone ileus.
F   Sigmoid volvulus.
G   Aortic dissection.
H   Consolidation of middle lobe of right lung.
I   Duodenal atresia.
J   Ovarian dermoid cyst.

Question 13. Signs and lesions

Characteristics of various lesions. Match the following.

Options

1   Skin colour normal.
2   Non-tender.
3   Fluctuance.
4   Mobile.
5   Pulsatile.
6   Compressible.
7   Punched out (square cut) edge.
8   Rolled edge.

Stems

A   Carotid body tumour.
B   Congenital dermoid cyst (non-ovarian).
C   Neuropathic ulcer.
D   Lipoma.
E   Arteriovenous malformation.
F   Basal cell carcinoma.
G   Histiocytoma.
H   Ganglion.

Question 14. Prostheses

Match the following.

Options

1   PTFE.
2   Homograft.
3   Xenograft.
4   Prolene.
5   Stainless steel.

6   Polyethylene.
7   Carbon.
8   Platinum.
9   Silicone.
10   Titanium.

Stems

A   Heart valve replacement.
B   Inguinal hernia repair.
C   Femoro-popliteal bypass.
D   Metacarpophalangeal joint.
E   Hip joint replacement.
F   Zygomatic fracture repair.
G   Stapedectomy.

Question 15. Prophylaxis

Match the following.

Options

1   Heparin.
2   *Haemophilus influenzae* type B vaccine.
3   Clopidogrel.
4   Dextran.
5   Aspirin.
6   N acetylcysteine.
7   Cefuroxime.
8   Meningococcal group C conjugate vaccine.
9   Metronidazole.
10   Tetanus toxoid booster.
11   Gentamicin.
12   Pneumatic compression.
13   TED stockings.
14   Amoxicillin.

Stems

A   Thromboprophylaxis prior to surgery.
B   Antibiotic prophylaxis pre-thyroid surgery.
C   Antibiotic prophylaxis pre-bowel surgery.
D   Renal protection prior to intravenous contrast.
E   Immunisation prior to elective splenectomy.
F   Dental procedures in patients with endocarditis or prosthetic heart valve.
G   Prophylaxis prior to urinary catheterisation in the presence of prosthesis.

Question 16. Eponymous signs

Match the following.

Options

1   Tinel's sign.
2   Trousseau's sign.
3   Acanthosis nigricans.
4   Rovsing's sign.
5   Phelan's sign.
6   Troisier's sign.
7   Horner's syndrome.
8   Chvostek's sign.
9   Virchow's node.
10   Virchow's triad.

Stems

A   Carpal tunnel syndrome.
B   Hypocalcaemia.
C   Appendicitis.
D   Pancoast's tumour.
E   Gastrointestinal tract malignancy.
F   Factors promoting thrombosis.

Question 17. Fluid and electrolytes

Match the following.

Options

1   Respiratory acidosis.
2   Respiratory alkalosis.
3   Hyperchloraemia.
4   Hypochloraemia.
5   Metabolic acidosis.
6   Metabolic alkalosis.
7   Hyponatraemia.
8   Hypernatraemia.

Stems

A   Persistent vomiting associated with pyloric stenosis.
B   High output ileostomy.
C   Diabetic ketoacidosis.
D   Chronic hyperventilation.
E   Breathing a gas mixture of 30% oxygen, 5% carbon dioxide and 65% nitrogen for 5 minutes.

Question 18. Nerve injuries

The following nerves may be damaged by trauma or at operation.

Options

1   Median nerve.
2   Ulnar nerve.
3   Mandibular branch of facial nerve.
4   Radial nerve.
5   Hypoglossal nerve.
6   Axillary nerve.
7   Common peroneal nerve.
8   Sympathetic chain.
9   Lingual nerve.
10   Sciatic nerve.

Stems

A   Fracture of humerus.
B   Fracture of fibula.
C   Carotid endarterectomy.
D   Excision of submandibular gland.
E   Brachial embolectomy.
F   Carpal tunnel decompression.

Question 19. Sterilisation procedures and prevention of transmission

Options

1   Effectively removes or destroys prions.
2   Effectively destroys virus particles.
3   Effectively destroys bacteria.
4   Can be used to sterilise delicate or perishable items.

Stems

A   Autoclave.
B   Manual washing and disinfection.
C   Glutaraldehyde.
D   Ethylene oxide.
E   Disposable single use items.
F   Gamma irradiation.
G   Moist heat (65°C for 30 minutes).
H   UV light.

Question 20. Anatomy of key points

Options

1   Lung.
2   Kidney.
3   Pleura.
4   Liver.
5   Inferior vena cava.
6   Diaphragm.
7   Appendix.
8   Fundus of gall bladder.
9   Portal vein.
10 Right renal vein.

Stems

A   Perpendicular and posterior stab wound below 12th rib to the right of the vertebral column will damage the following structures.

B   Pathology in the following structures may present with paraumbilical pain.

C   Anatomical relations of the right hepatic (colic) flexure.

D   Posterior relations of the second part of the duodenum include ...

E   Relations of the right adrenal gland.

Answer 1   A6, 7 & 8, B1, 3 & 6, C1, 2, 3 & 4, D1, 2, 3, 4 & 5,
                 E6, 8, (1, 3), F8 & 9, G8, H none

Management of wounds can be difficult. Clearly grossly contaminated
wounds need to be debrided, and closure either by delayed primary
closure or using an interrupted suture or clip to allow leakage of wound
fluid or pus. Drains may be placed to allow deeper tissues to drain
without development of static collections of fluid that could develop into
abscesses.

Answer 2   A5 & 8, B1, 4, 6 & 7, C2 & 3

Clear classification of wounds helps in decision-making. For example,
prophylactic antibiotics would be advisable to prevent wound infection
in clean contaminated wounds. Dirty wounds need debridement and
may be best managed by leaving open or by delayed primary closure.
Other common factors affecting wound healing include:
- Surgical technique
- Malnutrition
- Ischaemia
- Intercurrent illness
- Infection
- Previous irradiation
- Pre-operative nutrition
- Ehlers-Danlos syndrome
- Jaundice
- Impaired haemostasis with haematoma formation
- Steroid ingestion
- Diabetes mellitus

Answer 3   A4 & 6, B2, C1, & 4, D3, E(2), 4 & 5, F4 & 6, G4

GIA is the abbreviated name for Gastrointestinal Anastomosis stapler;
it can be used for constructing a variety of anastomoses in the gut.
Circular staplers are usually used most successfully in
oesophagogastric surgery and for low colorectal anastomoses. There is
no difference in leak rates between stapled and hand-sewn
anastomoses. Bowel preparation is advised for distal colonic resection
to reduce anastomotic leakage.

Answer 4   A5 & 8, B1, 2, 4, 5, 7 & 8, C1 & 5, D2, 4, 5 & 8, E2 & 5

In vascular surgery the use of prosthetic grafts is associated with increased risk of dehiscence with catastrophic limb or life-threatening effect.

Answer 5   A3 & 6, B3, C1, D3, E3, F4, 6 & 7, G3, H5, (6)

Minimally invasive techniques are becoming more popular and when carried out carefully can meet the demanding standards required for oncological surgery and even vascular surgery. This is an exciting time of change.

Answer 6   A6, B1, C none, D none, E5

Carbon dioxide insufflation is usually used for laparoscopy as it is very soluble; therefore, in the event of gas embolism due to insufflation into a blood vessel, there is a lower chance of major morbidity or death. Although the open 'Hassan' technique of trocar insertion reduces the risk of damage it does not prevent it completely.

Answer 7   A1, 2 & 8, B1, 3 & 9, C1 & 2, D10, E5, (6, 7), F5, 6 & 7, G1, 2 & 8

The history can help define the likely level of bowel obstruction. Associated problems such as nocturnal asthma may be the result of recurrent aspiration. Bile is unlikely to be in the vomitus unless the pylorus is incompetent which suggests that there is obstructed bowel distally. The absence of bile and presence of old food is suggestive of a failure of gastric emptying, this combined with a succussion splash is suggestive of gastric outlet vomiting. Faeculent vomiting is due to small bowel contents remaining static and becoming colonised with gut organisms, thus brown-stained, foul smelling vomit is produced. This is different to vomiting faeces; this indicates either a gastrocolic fistula or coprophagia.

Answer 8   A3, B3, 4, (5), C(3), D(3), E3, F7 & 8, G5, H1, 2, 3, 4, (5, 6), 7 & 8, I9, J1 & 2

The use of laparoscopic repair is recommended for bilateral or recurrent herniae. Until the procedure is clearly of benefit, those using the technique are advised to enter data onto a registry.

The development of mesh techniques has led to them being used extensively in many areas for repair of herniae. The mesh is a foreign body and there is a risk, albeit low, of prosthetic infection. When this occurs this can be disastrous, requiring removal of the mesh (if possible) and subsequent repair using alternative techniques.

Answer 9   A4 & 5, B6, C6, D8, E none

Answer 10   A none, B1, 2, 5, 6, 7, 9 & 12, C1, 3, 5, 6 & 12, D1, 4, 8, 10 & 13, E11 & 12, F6 & 12, G6, 11 & 12

Answer 11   A2, 3, 4 & 6, B2, 3, 4 & 6, C6, D4 & 6, E2, 3, 4 & 6, F2, 3, 4 & 6, G2, 5 & 6, H none

Blood transfusion should be avoided if at all possible, for many reasons including risk of transmission of viruses (Hepatitides, HIV and prions). There is likely to be a crisis in the availability of blood, in part due to the removal of existing and potential donors that have received blood products in the recent past, prior to screening for prions. All sensible measures should be taken to avoid transfusion, including careful surgical technique and special equipment, for instance, novel tools such as the Ligasure™ device.

Answer 12   A4, B1, C5, D6, E7 & 10, F9, G5, H8, I2, J11

Looser's zone is a transverse lucent band seen in bones affected by osteomalacia; it is often symmetrical.

Answer 13   A1, 2 & 5, B1, 2 & 3, C2 & 7, D1, 2 & 3, E2 & 6, F2 & 8, G2, H1, 2 & 3

Examination of a lesion must record the position, colour, temperature, tenderness, size and shape, followed by an appreciation of the base, edge, depth, discharge, surrounding tissues and anylocallymphadenopathy.

There are 5 types of ulcer edge:

1. A sloping edge (suggests healing, eg. venous ulcer).
2. A punched out edge (follows rapid death and skin loss, eg. diabetes, neuropathic ulcer).
3. An undermined edge (seen when infection affects the tissues, eg. pressure necrosis of TB).
4. An everted edge (tissue on the edge is rapidly growing, eg. squamous cell cancer).
5. A rolled edge (slow growth of tissues in the edge of the ulcer, eg. basal cell cancer).

Answer 14   A2, 3 & 7, B4, C1, 2 & 3, D6 & 9, E5 & 6, F8 & 10, G1, 2 & 8

Answer 15   A1, 11 & 13, B none, C7, 9 & 11, D6, E2 & 8, F11 & 14, G11

The incidence of DVT is reduced by the use of intermittent pneumatic compression boots, graduated compression (TED) stockings and heparin (unfractionated or low molecular weight).

Reference to current guidelines in the British National Formulary is recommended with respect to antibacterial therapy.

Answer 16   A1 & 5, B2 & 8, C4, D7, E6 & 9, F10

Tinel's sign is percussion over the flexor aspect of the wrist, at the flexor retinaculum. This reproduces tingling or an electric shock sensation in the sensory territory of median nerve, indicating compression of the median nerve in the carpal tunnel.

Phelan's sign requires forced flexion of the wrist. In cases of carpal tunnel syndrome, paraesthesia is experienced in the territory of the median nerve.

Rovsing's sign is pressure in the left iliac fossa causing pain in the right iliac fossa; this is indicative of appendicitis.

Virchow's triad is used to describe factors that predispose to thrombosis, namely hypercoagulability of the blood, abnormality of the vessel wall or reduction in flow/stasis of the blood.

Troisier's sign is the presence of a lymph node in the left supraclavicular fossa, (i.e. Virchow's node); this is often associated with a malignancy of the GI tract, usually the stomach. This is due to lymphatic drainage of the GI tract via the thoracic duct.

Acanthosis nigricans is hyperpigmentation of the axilla; it is associated with gastric neoplasm.

Chvostek's sign is seen in tetany; tapping the facial nerve results in twitching of the facial muscles. This is indicative of hypocalcaemia.

Trousseau's phenomenon is a sign of latent tetany. Spasm of the hand and wrist with adduction of the thumb, bunching of the fingers and flexion of the wrist, which is produced by compression of the forearm, in subjects having undue neuromuscular excitability as a result of deficiency in ionised calcium.

Horner's syndrome is mild enophthalmos, miosis and ptosis ipsilaterally with decreased skin sweating. It is due to interference with the cervical sympathetic fibres on the affected side possibly secondary to a tumour of the lung (Pancoast's tumour).

Answer 17   A4, 6 & 7, B7, C5, D2, E1

Answer 18   A2, 4 & 6, B7, C3, 5 & 8, D3 & 9, E1, F1

Answer 19   A2 & 3, B4, C2 & 3, D2, 3, & 4, E none, F2, 3, 4,
                  G none, H none

Autoclave is the usual method of sterilising surgical instruments, dressings and culture media. In high vacuum autoclaves >98% of air is removed and rapid sterilisation is possible (for example, 3 minutes, 134°C and 200 kPa).

UV light has powerful germicidal properties but its powers of penetration are so slight that its practical usefulness is limited.

Ionising gamma radiations (cobalt 60 and caesium 137) are very penetrating and can be used to sterilise articles up to 0.5m thick (for example, heat sensitive prepared articles including bone grafts, surgical sutures, syringes and catheters).

Ethylene oxide diffuses rapidly thought paper, fabrics and plastics. It can be used for sterilising delicate instruments.

Prions, the likely cause of the human variant CJD, cannot be destroyed by traditional methods. They have been identified in tonsil specimens and appendices. The current approach in ENT surgery is to use disposable instruments for tonsillectomy. No such recommendation exists currently for appendicectomy.

Answer 20   A2, 3 & 5, B7, C2, 4 & 8, D2 & 10, E2, 4, 5 & 6

It is important to remember when dealing with a stabbing case all the possible structures related to the entry and exit wounds. The posterior attachment of the pleura crosses the 12th rib and passes horizontally to the lower border of the 12th thoracic vertebra. This triangle of pleura lies behind the upper pole of the kidney. The lower limit of the lung is the 10th rib. The lower border of the liver lies at the upper border of the 12th rib.

The paraumbilical region is supplied by the T10 spinal nerve and it is via referred pain from the appendix, small bowel and testes that discomfort is experienced in this area.

The boundaries of the hepatic flexure are the renal fascia, right lobe of the liver, right adrenal gland and second part of the duodenum.

The hilum of the right kidney with the renal vein and artery lie behind the second part of the duodenum. The portal vein lies behind the pancreas and the first part of the duodenum.

Chapter 2

Anaesthetics

Aidan Byrne, MD MRCP FRCA

Consultant Anaesthetist, Morriston Hospital, Swansea, UK

For all questions each option may be used once, more than once or not at all.

Question 1. Admission to the ITU

What is likely to be the reason for admitting the following patients to an ITU?

Options

1   Intensive monitoring.
2   Organ failure.
3   Intensive nursing care.
4   Ventilation.
5   Lowered Glasgow Coma Score.
6   Epidural anaesthesia.

Stems

A   Postoperative, clipping of an intracranial aneurysm.
B   Severe closed head injury.
C   Opiate overdose.
D   60% second degree burns.
E   Severe sepsis.

Question 2. Sedatives

The following sedatives are likely to be chosen.

Options

1   Lack of metabolites.
2   Able to be given by inhalation.
3   Cheap.
4   Profound amnesia.
5   Ultra short duration of action, with cough suppression.
6   The need to avoid coughing.

Stems

A   Propofol.
B   Isoflurane.
C   Neuromuscular blocker.
D   Benzodiazepine.
E   Remifentanil.

Question 3. Hypoxia

In the following conditions, the hypoxia is mainly caused by:

Options

1   Hypoventilation.
2   V/Q mismatch.
3   Shunt.
4   Pulmonary oedema.
5   Airway obstruction.
6   Lowered barometric pressure.

Stems

A   Guillian-Barre.
B   Lung trauma.
C   Left ventricular failure.
D   Acute epiglottitis.
E   Congenital cyanotic heart disease.

Question 4. Severity scoring systems

Options

1   Glasgow Coma Score.
2   Therapeutic Intervention Scoring System.
3   APACHE2.
4   Mortality prediction models.

Stems

A   Is specific for a single organ system.
B   Is designed to measure the workload of staff.
C   Is dependent on the style of patient management.
D   Can easily be calculated without the use of computers.
E   Requires detailed information on a range of physiological measures.

Question 5. Complications of tracheal intubation

Options

1   Tracheal stenosis.
2   Severity of hypertensive response.
3   Risk of oesophageal intubation.
4   Risk of aspiration of gastric contents.
5   Dislocation of an arytenoid cartilage.
6   Laryngeal nerve damage.

Stems

A   Is reduced by cricoid pressure.
B   Is reduced by prior administration of an opioid.
C   Is a late complication.
D   Is reduced by a rapid sequence induction.
E   Is increased by a larger diameter tracheal tube.

Question 6. Ventilation

The following are true of modes of ventilation.

Options

1   Volume controlled.
2   Pressure controlled.
3   Positive End Expiratory Pressure.
4   Continuous positive airway pressure.
5   High frequency ventilation.
6   High frequency jet ventilation.

Stems

A   Involves small tidal volumes delivered at rates of 60-150 cycles per minute.
B   Tidal volume will change if the patient's abdomen distends.
C   Is used with spontaneously breathing patients.
D   Delivers a relatively large fixed volume of gas into the lungs.
E   Tidal volume will not change if the patient's abdomen distends.

Question 7. Pathology

Link the following physiological problem to the pathology.

Options

1   Hypovolaemia.
2   Obstructed venous return.
3   Pump failure.
4   Low systemic vascular resistance.
5   Obstructed arterial flow.

Stems

A   Septic shock.
B   Pericardial effusion.
C   Aortic coarctation
D   Hypertrophic obstructive cardiomyopathy (HOCM).
E   Complete heart block.

Question 8. Measurement of arterial blood gases

Options

1   Is measured by a blood gas analyser and affects the alveolar partial pressure of oxygen.
2   Is measured by a blood gas analyser and doesn't affect the alveolar partial pressure of oxygen.
3   Is calculated by a blood gas analyser and doesn't affect the alveolar partial pressure of oxygen.
4   Is calculated by a blood gas analyser and affects the alveolar partial pressure of oxygen.
5   Is not usually part of a blood gas estimation but affects the alveolar partial pressure of oxygen.
6   Is not usually part of a blood gas estimation and doesn't affect the alveolar partial pressure of oxygen.

Stems

A   Barometric pressure.
B   Base deficit.
C PaO_2.
D   pH.
E   Haemoglobin concentration.

Question 9. Oxygen delivery

For a patient who starts with a haemoglobin of 16g/dL, a cardiac output of 5L/min and an oxygen saturation of 100%, the oxygen delivery, as a percentage of the original value, will fall to:

Options

1   80%.
2   75%.
3   50%.
4   25%.
5   12.5%.
6   10%.
7   5%.

Stems

A   A haemoglobin of 8g/dL, cardiac output of 5L/min and oxygen saturation of 100%.
B   A haemoglobin of 16g/dL, cardiac output of 5L/min and oxygen saturation of 50%.
C   A haemoglobin of 8g/dL, cardiac output of 2.5L/min and oxygen saturation of 50%.
D   A haemoglobin of 16g/dL, cardiac output of 5L/min and oxygen saturation of 50%.
E   A haemoglobin of 8g/dL, cardiac output of 5L/min and oxygen saturation of 50%.

Question 10. Cardiac output

The following methods of measuring cardiac output use the principle of:

Options

1   Heating blood.
2   Cooling blood.
3   Measuring the velocity of red cells.
4   Measuring the concentration of a marker.
5   Measuring changes in the conductivity of the thorax.
6   Measuring changes in the movement of the body.

Stems

A   Impedance cardiography.
B   Continuous thermodilution.
C   Lithium dilution.
D   Oesphageal doppler.
E   Intermittent cardiac output.

Question 11. Inotropes

The following inotropes are best used to cause:

Options

1   Vasoconstriction.
2   Increased cardiac output.
3   Vasoconstriction and increased cardiac output.
4   Increased cardiac output and dose-dependant effects of vasculature.
5   Vasodilation.
6   Vasodilation and increased cardiac output.
7   None of the above.

Stems

A   Adrenaline.
B   Enoxiparin.
C   Noradrenaline.
D   Dopamine.
E   Milrinone.

Question 12. Brain stem death

The following are associated with the diagnosis of:

Options

1   Brain stem death.
2   Normal function.
3   Not relevant to brain stem death testing.

Stems

A   Pupillary constriction to a direct light stimulus.
B   No respiratory effort after $PaCO_2$ risen to 4.7 Kpa.
C   Absent abdominal reflexes.
D   Absent gag reflex.
E   Arm extension to peripheral nerve stimulation.

Question 13. Parenteral nutrition

The following are linked in parenteral nutrition.

Options

1 Fatty liver.
2 Pancreatitis.
3 Hyperglycaemia.
4 Hyperkalaemia.
5 Hyponatremia.
6 Pink blood samples.
7 Sepsis.

Stems

A Glucose containing solutions.
B Lipid containing solutions.
C Electrolyte-free solutions.
D Long-term use of parenteral nutrition with 65% of calories provided by glucose.
E Non-tunnelled catheters.

Question 14. Central venous cannulation

Complications of central venous cannulation are usually due to:

Options

1 Needle insertion.
2 Wire insertion.
3 Injection of local anaesthetic.
4 Radiation from screening.
5 Presence of catheter.

Stems

A Arrythmias.
B Pneumothorax.
C Arterial bleeding.
D Thrombosis.
E Infection.

Answer 1   A1, B1, 4 & 5, C4, D3, E1, 2, 3 & 4

The management of an individual patient usually depends on a single critical factor. In the case of head injuries it is the severity of the injury (measured by GCS), for sepsis it is the onset of multi-organ failure, for burns patients it is the need for frequent dressing changes, analgesia and general nursing care.

Answer 2   A1, B1, 2 & 4, C6, D4, E1, 5 & 6

Any sedative has some properties which make it useful. Propofol is short acting, but does not suppress the cough reflex.

Answer 3   A1, B2, C4, D5, E3

Guillian-Barre syndrome causes muscle weakness and hypoventilation. Lung trauma usually leads to a loss of regulation in the lung vasculature and hence V/Q mismatch. The shunt of congenital heart disease leads to the ineffectiveness of oxygen therapy.

Answer 4   A1, B2, C2, D1, E3 & 4

TISS measures the number and type of interventions used on the ITU, but is very dependent on the policies of the unit. The more aggressive the unit, the higher the scores will be for the same patient mix. All the scores, except the GCS, require the data to be entered onto computers to make the calculations on a daily basis. APACHE 2 in particular can only be calculated within the commercially available programme.

Answer 5   A4, B2, C1, D4, E5

Aspiration is reduced by using cricoid pressure and a rapid sequence intubation technique, but this leads to more haemodynamic instability.

Answer 6   A5, B2, C4, D1, E1

In volume control, a fixed volume is pushed in at inspiration, so pressure varies. In pressure control a fixed pressure is applied, so volume varies. PEEP is used in ventilated patients. The equivalent technique of keeping a small pressure applied to the lungs throughout the respiratory cycle is known as CPAP (continuous positive airway pressure).

Answer 7   A1 & 4, B3, C5, D5, E3

Sepsis causes a drop in sytemic vascular resistance and can be associated with either hypo- or hypervolaemia. While aortic stenosis and HOCM are associated with obstruction of flow, this occurs within the heart, leading to pump failure.

Answer 8   A5, B3, C1, D2, E2

A blood gas analyser generally measures pH, and the partial pressure of oxygen and carbon dioxide. The base deficit is a measure of metabolic acidosis, but is calculated from other values. The barometric pressure is needed to calculate the inspired partial pressure of oxygen by multiplying it with the inspired fraction of oxygen (usually 21%).

Answer 9   A3, B3, C5, D3, E4

Oxygen delivery is a product of cardiac output, haemoglobin concentration and saturation. Halving each reduces oxygen delivery to one eighth of its original value.

Answer 10   A5, B1, C4, D3, E2

Answer 11   A3, B7, C1, D4, E6

Answer 12   A2, B1, C3, D1, E3

Answer 13   A1 & 3, B2 & 6, C5, D1, E7

Lipid-containing TPN commonly causes increased fat in the blood (lipaemia) which makes any blood samples look pink. Fatty liver is rarely seen now, but was common before lipid-based TPN became available. Tunnelling catheters significantly reduces the infection rate.

Answer 14   A2 & 5, B1, C1, D5, E5

Insertion of a needle into the neck commonly causes bleeding and less commonly pneumothorax. Insertion of a Seldinger wire almost invariably causes arrythmias if inserted into the atria. The doses of local anaesthetic and radiation used rarely cause problems.

Chapter 3

Intensive care

Sean Dwyer, MB BS FRCA

Consultant Anaesthetist, Morriston Hospital, Swansea, UK

For all questions each option may be used once, more than once or not at all.

Question 1. Chest pain

For a patient with sudden onset chest pain 8hrs post THR, match the most appropriate pairs.

Options

1   ECG.
2   CXR.
3   V/Q scan.
4   ABG.
5   INR.

Stems

A   First.
B   Second.
C   Third.
D   Fourth.
E   Not indicated.

Question 2. Blood gas analysis

For a postoperative patient on 40% oxygen by facemask, match the following.

Options

1 PaO_2 9.0 KPa.
2 $PaCO_2$ 6.0 KPa.
3 pH 7.2.
4 B.E. -6.
5 Lactate 3.0.

Stems

A Indicates hypoperfusion.
B Indicates metabolic acidosis.
C Indicates respiratory acidosis.
D Indicates hypoxia.
E Indicates respiratory depression.

Question 3. Head injury

In a patient with a single dilated pupil and a GCS of 6, match the following.

Options

1 CT scan head.
2 Neuro observations.
3 Intubation.
4 ABG.
5 IV mannitol.

Stems

A First.
B Second.
C Third.
D Fourth.
E Fifth.

Question 4. Trauma

A 20-year-old male with no coexisting pathology presents post RTA. He withdraws from painful stimulus, vocalises inappropriately and does not open his eyes. He has a pulse of 160bpm and a blood pressure of 90/60mmHg. Match the following.

Options

1 GCS scoring.
2 Intubation and ventilation.
3 Intravenous access.
4 Volume resuscitation.

Stems

A Should occur as rapidly as possible within the first hour from time of injury.
B Is not appropriate for the given scenario.
C If performed could put the patient at greater risk.
D Should be delayed until senior help is available.
E Should be delayed until the precise nature of the injury is known.

Question 5. Organ donation

In a patient being considered for organ donation, match the following statements appropriately.

Options

1 Brain stem death tests.
2 Temperature of 34.9 Celsius.
3 pH 7.1.
4 Apnoeic coma requiring ventilation.
5 Irreversible brain damage of known cause.

Stems

A Are preconditions for donation.
B Are exclusions for donation.
C Neither of the above.

Question 6. Cardiovascular physiology

Match the following statements appropriately.

Options

1   Cardiac output.
2   Oxygen delivery.
3   Blood pressure.
4   Systemic vascular resistance.

Stems

A   A function of cardiac output and systemic vascular resistance.
B   Mean arterial pressure - central venous pressure x 79.9/cardiac output.
C   Heart rate x stroke volume.
D $CI \times CaO_2 \times 10$.

Question 7. Pre-operative assessment

In patients over the age of 65 presenting for urgent major surgery, match the stems appropriately.

Options

1   Newly diagnosed hypertension.
2   Newly diagnosed diabetes.
3   Poorly controlled asthma.
4   Myocardial infarction 6 months previously.
5   History of DVT after surgery in the past.

Stems

A   Should be controlled as an inpatient prior to surgery.
B   Should be controlled as an outpatient prior to surgery.
C   Requires no further investigation so long as initial management was complete.

Question 8. Differential diagnosis

A tachypnoeic, hypotensive patient with distended neck veins.

Options

1   Tension pneumothorax.
2   Myocardial infarction.
3   Cardiac tamponade.
4   Hypovolaemic shock.
5   Pulmonary embolus.

Stems

A   Likely diagnosis.
B   Unlikely diagnosis.
C   Await results of investigation prior to treatment.
D   CXR is mandatory prior to treatment.

Question 9. Complications

The following can be complications of:

Options

1   Ventricular tachycardia.
2   Right atrial perforation.
3   Pneumothorax.
4   Pulmonary infarction.
5   Left atrial perforation.

Stems

A   Internal jugular lines.
B   Pulmonary artery catheters.
C   Subclavian lines.

Question 10. Intracranial pressure and cerebral blood flow

Options

1 Hyperventilation.
2 Trendelenberg position.
3 Induced hypotension.
4 General anaesthesia.
5 Intravenous mannitol.

Stems

A Decreases ICP.
B Increases ICP.
C Decreases CBF.
D Increases CBF.

Question 11. Respiratory physiology

Options

1 Oxygen hunger.
2 Increased dead space.
3 Increased V/Q mismatch.
4 Hypoventilation.
5 Decreased V/Q mismatch.

Stems

A Chemoreceptor response.
B Consequent to hypoxic pulmonary artery vasoconstriction.
C Leads to a further deterioration in gas exchange.
D Does not occur.

Question 12. Tracheal intubation

Options

1 Airway protection.
2 Airway patency.
3 Paralysis.
4 Duration of ventilation.
5 Hypoxia.

Stems

A An indication for intubation.
B Not an indication for intubation.

Question 13. Invasive monitoring

Indications of the following can be obtained from observation of which of the following?

Options

1 Myocardial contractility.
2 Circulating volume.
3 Systemic vascular resistance (SVR).
4 Mitral regurgitation (MR).
5 Aortic regurgitation (AR).

Stems

A Arterial waveform.
B Central venous pressure.
C Pulmonary artery waveform.

Question 14. Prioritising intervention

In a patient with peritonitis and severe documented coronary artery disease (CAD) requiring emergency laparotomy.

Options

1   Oxygen by facemask.
2   Intravenous access and fluid resuscitation.
3   Analgesia.
4   Coronary angiography.
5   Central venous pressure (CVP) measurement.

Stems

A   First.
B   Second.
C   Third.
D   Fourth.
E   Fifth.

Question 15. Diagnosis

Match the most likely with the given scenarios.

Options

1   PE.
2   MI.
3   Pneumonia.
4   Hypovolaemia.
5   Opioid analgesia.

Stems

A   60-year-old man 8 hours post-AAA repair, tachycardic, hypotensive, peripherally vasoconstricted.

B   87-year-old female 24 hours post-DHS, confused, hypotensive, bradypnoeic, with a falling GCS.

C   54-year-old man 96 hours post-laparotomy on PCA. Tachypnoeic, pyrexial, hypotensive.

D   28-year-old man 12 hours post-tibial nailing, tachypnoeic, hypotensive, in distress.

E   60-year-old female with a history of hypertension, 72 hours post-TAH, hypotensive, tachypnoeic, coarse creps throughout the chest on auscultation.

Question 16. Circulating volume

In loss of circulating volume which of the following corresponds to the appropriate % loss of circulating volume?

Options

1   Tachycardia >120 bpm.
2   Coma.
3   Tachycardia with severe hypotension.
4   Mild tachycardia with oliguria.
5   Thirst and vasoconstriction.

Stems

A   10%.
B   20%.
C   30%.
D   40%.
E   50%.

Question 17. Ionic imbalance

Concerning sodium and potassium balance, the following can cause:

Options

1   Salt restriction.
2   Glycine irrigation.
3   Dehydration.
4   GI fluid sequestration.
5   Renal failure.

Stems

A   Hyponatraemia.
B   Hypernatraemia.
C   Hypokalaemia.
D   Hyperkalaemia.

Question 18. Ionic imbalance

Which of the following conditions can be associated with which ionic imbalance/s?

Options

1   Hypertension.
2   Tented T waves.
3   Convulsions.
4   Multiple premature ventricular contractions.

Stems

A   Hypokalaemia.
B   Hyponatraemia.
C   Hyperkalaemia.
D   Hypocalcaemia.

Question 19. Blood gases

Match the following blood gas values with the appropriate statement/s.

Options

1   pH 7.4.
2   $PaCO_2$ 5.3 KPa.
3   PaO_2 12 KPa.
4   HCO_3 25mEq/l.
5   BE 0.

Stems

A   Within normal range.
B   Above normal range.
C   Below normal range.

Question 20. Modes of ventilation

Options

1   Positive end expiratory pressure.
2   Pressure controlled ventilation.
3   Intermittent positive pressure ventilation.
4   Synchronised intermittent mandatory ventilation.

Stems

A   Optimises V/Q matching.
B   Most common ventilatory mode in the operating theatre.
C   Weaning mode of ventilation.
D   Avoids barotraumas in ventilation.

Question 21. Postoperative aspiration

Aspiration of gastric contents in the immediate postoperative period.

Options

1   Immediate intubation and ventilation.
2   Prophylactic antibiotic cover.
3   Admission to intensive care.
4   Regular observation prior to specific therapy.

Stems

A   Is mandatory.
B   Is advisable.
C   Is not necessary unless clinically indicated.

Question 22. Complications

Match the following appropriately.

Options

1   Acute pancreatitis.
2   Road traffic accident.
3   Sepsis.
4   Massive blood transfusion.
5   Cardiopulmonary bypass.

Stems

A   Is associated with ALI (acute lung injury).
B   Is not associated with ALI.
C   Is associated with ARF (acute renal failure).
D   Is not associated with ARF.

Question 23. Invasive monitoring

Match the following monitoring devices with the parameters that they can play a part in measuring or deriving.

Options

1   PA catheter.
2   Urinary catheter.
3   Nasopharyngeal thermistor.
4   Blood gas analyser.
5   Indwelling arterial cannula.

Stems

A   Core temperature.
B   Oxygen delivery.
C   Cardiac output.
D   Systemic vascular resistance.
E   Oxygen consumption.

Question 24. Postoperative complications

Match the most likely cause for the given clinical scenario in a 72-year-old man 36 hours post-bowel resection.

Options

1   Hypertensive, raised creatinine, oliguric with a normal pulse rate.
2   Hypotensive, tachycardic, raised creatinine and oliguria.
3   Hypotensive, tachycardic, normal urine output, raised urea, normal creatinine.
4   Hypertensive, tachycardic, anuric, raised creatinine, distended bladder.

Stems

A   Acute bleed into GI tract.
B   Pre-renal failure.
C   Intrinsic renal failure.
D   Post-renal failure

Question 25. Blood gases

Match the blood gases with the conditions.

Options

1   pH 7.10, PaO_2 5.1 KPa, $PaCO_2$ 7.4 KPa, HCO_3 25.0 meq/l, be
    - 1.0.
2   pH 7.38, PaO_2 6.0 KPa, $PaCO_2$ 8.2 KPa, HCO_3 35.0 meq/l, be
    + 6.0.
3   pH 7.2, PaO_2 13.0 KPa, $PaCO_2$ 3.2 KPa, HCO_3 15.0 meq/l, be
    - 6.0.

Stems

A   Acute asthma.
B   Rebreathing from a closed circuit.
C   Hypoxic drive.
D   Hypoperfusion.
E   Reperfusion.

Question 26. Rescuscitation

A patient is found collapsed apnoeic and pulseless 3 hours postoperatively. In what order should intervention occur?

Options

1   DC cardioversion.
2   Bag and mask ventilation.
3   External cardiac massage.
4   Intubation.
5   Peripheral venous access.

Stems

A   First.
B   Second.
C   Third.
D   Fourth.
E   Fifth.

Answer 1   A1, B2, C4, D3, E5

The important differential diagnoses are pulmonary embolus (PE) or myocardial ischaemia and both should be rapidly diagnosed or excluded and appropriate treatment commenced as soon as possible to limit further damage. An ECG can be quickly performed whilst awaiting mobile CXR. An ABG performed and rapidly analysed can give valuable information in relation to oxygen delivery. A V/Q scan is diagnostic for PE and can be performed later if indicated; an INR in a non-anticoagulated patient is of little use.

Answer 2   A3, 4, & 5, B3, 4 & 5, C2 & 3, D1, E2, 3, 4 & 5

Hypoperfusion allows tissue hypoxia to develop with anaerobic metabolism and lactate production. This leads to a fall in pH, raised lactate and a base deficit and is a metabolic acidosis. A raised $PaCO_2$ causes an increase in carbonic acid and hence a fall in pH. A PaO_2 of only 9.0 on supplemental oxygen is relatively hypoxic whilst a raised $PaCO_2$ in the presence of a metabolic acidosis indicates respiratory depression.

Answer 3   A2, B3, C4, D5, E1

In such a patient the most likely pathology is a rising ICP. Institution of regular neuro observations gives a baseline from which further observations will show the results of any intervention. The airway is at risk and must be secured. This will consequently allow manipulation of $PaCO_2$ and hence ICP. Regular ABG analysis will allow assessment of oxygen content, $PaCO_2$, Hct, and blood sugar. IV mannitol will cause an acute drop in UCP if needed whilst awaiting a CT scan.

Answer 4   A1, 2, 3 & 4, B, C, D & E none.

In a healthy young man a heart rate of 160bpm with any degree of hypotension indicates decompensation in the face of profound hypovolaemia. Irrespective of the cause of his GCS of 6 he should have his airway secured, oxygen delivery assured and circulating volume rapidly restored if he is to survive. All the interventions mentioned should be considered as basic to all clinicians involved in the care of trauma victims.

Answer 5   A1, 4 & 5, B2 & 3, C none

Answer 6   A3, B4, C1, D2

Answer 7   A1, 2 & 3, B none, C4 & 5

Uncontrolled hypertension, diabetes and asthma will all significantly increase the morbidity and mortality associated with major surgery. As surgery is urgent then inpatient control will be most rapid and allow surgery to commence at the earliest possible time, whereas outpatient control will cause unacceptable delay. A patient with an MI 6 months previously will be at the same risk as anyone with a previous infarct, and DVT postoperatively in the past requires no special pre-operative consideration.

Answer 8   A1, 2, 3 & 5, B4, C & D none

Neck veins will not be distended in hypovolaemic shock. All the other conditions are immediately life-threatening when severe enough to cause these signs and symptoms, and require rapid clinical diagnosis and prompt treatment.

Answer 9   A1, 2 & 3, B1, 2, 3 & 4, C1, 2 & 3

Answer 10   A1, 3 & 5, B2 & 4, C3, D4

Answer 11   A1, B3, C3, D4 & 5

Hypovolaemia causes hypoperfusion, anaerobic metabolism and lactic acidosis with consequent compensatory hyperventilation. Relative hypoxia causes hypoxic pulmonary artery vasoconstriction worsening gas exchange by increasing V/Q mismatch.

Answer 12   A1 & 3, B2, 4 & 5

A cuffed ET tube will protect the airway from soiling from above or below. A paralysed patient will require intubation to allow effective ventilation to occur in the first instance. A patent airway can be maintained without intubation and intubation does nothing to correct hypoxia. Patients can be ventilated for very long times in cuirasse devices without being intubated.

Answer 13   A1, 2, 3 & 5, B2, C4

The upstroke of the arterial waveform gives an indication of myocardial contractility, the volume under the curve and the presence or absence of a respiratory swing, an indication of circulating volume and the gradient of the down stroke, an indication of SVR. An obviously wide pulse pressure with late or absent dichrotic notch is indicative of AR whilst M waves on the pulmonary artery waveform are indicative of MR.

Answer 14   A1, B2, C3, D5, E none

Pain, hypovolaemia and tachycardia all combine to increase myocardial oxygen demand. In the face of stenotic CAD this is likely to precipitate ischaemia greatly increasing morbidity and mortality. Care should be taken with fluid resuscitation as there is a risk of precipitating LVF. Optimally, fluid should be given whilst measuring the CVP.

Answer 15   A4, B5, C3, D2, E1

Note that all patients are hypotensive and require rapid intervention in what are all life-threatening conditions. Pre-morbid states, time postop and nature of the condition must be used to direct simple investigation and rapid management. The wrong diagnosis can lead to inappropriate management which could in itself be fatal.

Answer 16   A5, B4, C1, D3, E2

Answer 17   A1 & 2, B3 & 5, C4, D5

Answer 18   A4, B1 & 3, C2, D none

Answer 19   A1, 2, 3, 4 & 5, B none, C none

This is a normal blood gas.

Answer 20   A1, B3, C4, D2

Positive End Expiratory Pressure (PEEP) keeps alveoli open at the end of expiration that would otherwise collapse as closing volume was reached. This allows these alveoli to take part in gas exchange and therefore optimises V/Q matching.

Pressure controlled ventilation (PCV) limits the inspiratory pressure and so decreases the likelihood of pressure induced damage on the lung. In this mode, tidal volume becomes dependent on the set pressure, the inspiratory flow rate and time, and the lung compliance.

Synchronised Intermittent Mandatory Ventilation (SIMV) allows spontaneous assisted breaths to be taken between set ventilated breaths and allows gradual weaning from the ventilator.

Intermittent Positive Pressure Ventilation (IPPV) allows tidal volume and respiratory rate to be set and attained irrespective of the inspiratory pressure.

Answer 21   A4, B2, C1 & 3

The harmful effects of aspiration of gastric contents are determined by the nature of the contents (eg. solid or liquid), the volume aspirated and the pH of the aspirate. The effects can range from none to complete airway obstruction but there is usually some degree of pneumonitis with or without secondary bacterial infection. Close and regular observation will determine the initial degree of damage, its course and severity. This in turn will direct therapy.

Answer 22   A1, 2, 3, 4 & 5, B none, C1, 2, 3, 4 & 5, D none

Answer 23   A1, 2 & 3, B1 & 4, C1, D1 & 5, E1 & 4

PA catheters have a thermistor at the end to allow measurement of PA blood temp. Temperature probes on bladder catheters or nasopharyngeal probes also give core temperature readings. Oxygen content, delivery and consumption can be estimated with data obtained from cardiac output, SpO_2, SVO_2, Hct and cardiac output. A PA catheter can measure CO and with MAP and other measured variables, allow estimation of SVR.

Answer 24   A3, B2, C1, D4

The raised urea with normal creatinine in the face of signs of hypovolaemia, indicate GI bleeding with subsequent absorption of haemoglobin in the gut.

Signs of hypovolaemia with oliguria and raised creatinine indicate decreased renal perfusion.

Intrinsic renal failure is associated with hypertension and a normal pulse, whereas the hypertension associated with the distress of bladder outflow obstruction will be accompanied by a tachycardia.

Answer 25   A1, B1, C2, D3, E3

In acute severe asthma the development of a respiratory acidosis in the face of hypoxia is a very worrying state requiring rapid treatment. The same gases can be obtained from rebreathing without CO_2 absorption.

A compensated respiratory acidosis with associated hypoxia shows that a raised CO_2 is no longer the principal drive to respiration.

An increased production of lactate will give a metabolic acidosis. This can present either as a consequence of hypoperfusion and anaerobic metabolism or the reperfusion of areas left absolutely or relatively ischaemic.

Answer 26   A2, B3, C4, D5, E1

Airway and breathing first prior to establishment of rudimentary circulation, then securing the airway prior to establishing a means of pharmacological circulatory support, and then cardioversion if indicated.

Chapter 4

Vascular surgery

Louis J Fligelstone, MB BCh MD FRCS(Eng) FRCS(Gen)
Consultant Surgeon, Morriston Hospital, Swansea, UK
Alun H Davies, MA DM FRCS
Reader in Surgery and Consultant Surgeon,
Imperial College School of Medicine, Charing Cross Hospital, London, UK

For all questions each option may be used once, more than once or not at all.

Question 1. Intermittent claudication

Patients presenting with pain in their legs on exercise.

Options

1   Immediate onset.
2   Relieved by rest.
3   Relieved by sitting.
4   Worse climbing stairs.
5   Associated with lying flat.
6   Variable distance.
7   Worse on inclines.
8   Paraesthesia.
9   Affects ankle.
10 Radiates into foot.
11 Worse in the morning.
12 Pain radiates to knee.
13 Pain deep in the hip.

Stems

A   Intermittent claudication.
B   Sciatica.
C   Spinal claudication.
D   Osteoarthritis of hip.
E   Hammer toes.

Question 2. Claudication

The following vascular abnormality may cause the following symptoms.

Options

1   Pain in buttocks and thighs.
2   Pain in thigh and calf.
3   Pain in calf muscles.
4   Male impotence.
5   Pain in the toes.
6   Pain disturbing sleep.
7   Calf pain in bed.

Stems

A   Isolated superficial femoral artery occlusion.
B   External iliac occlusion.
C   Common iliac occlusion.
D   Isolated posterior tibial 25% stenosis.

Question 3. Carotid disease

You are the SHO in the vascular clinic.

Options

1   Full blood count.
2   Listen for a right carotid bruit.
3   Duplex ultrasound of superficial femoral artery.
4   Ankle brachial pressure index.
5   Duplex ultrasound of carotid arteries.
6   Reassure him and arrange review in 3 months.
7   Fasting lipids.
8   Homocysteine levels.
9   Angiography.
10   Magnetic resonance scan.
11   Review notes.
12   Thrombophilia screen.
13   Aortic ultrasound.

Stems

A   72-year-old male patient attends the outpatient for review of his intermittent claudication.

B   65-year-old male patient attends the outpatient for review of his intermittent claudication but complains that he has had transient weakness of his right leg, lasting for one hour 2 days ago.

C   45-year-old man complains of leg pain on exertion, steadily deteriorating over 6 months.

D   70-year-old man with asymptomatic left carotid bruit.

E   20-year-old woman with asymptomatic varicose veins.

Question 4. Carotid disease

Symptoms and lesions.

Options

1 Right amaurosis fugax.
2 Dizziness.
3 Unsteady gait.
4 Diplopia.
5 Transient weakness of right upper limb.
6 Dysphasia.
7 Left homonomous hemianopia.
8 Pin-point pupils and gross hypertension.

Stems

A Vertebrobasilar symptoms.
B Left carotid stenosis.
C Right carotid stenosis.
D Vertigo.
E Subclavian steal syndrome.
F Brainstem infarct.

Question 5. Investigation of certain conditions

The following provides a definite diagnosis in the conditions listed.

Options

1 Duplex ultrasound scan.
2 CT scan.
3 Magnetic resonance scan.
4 Scintigraphy.
5 Digital subtraction angiography.

Stems

A   Carotid body tumour.
B   Carotid stenosis.
C   Abdominal aortic aneurysm.
D   Peripheral arterial lesions.
E   Aortic occlusion.
F   Venous thrombosis.

Question 6. Vascular diseases

Options

1   5-7% of middle-aged to elderly people suffer symptoms from this.
2   20% of the population suffer symptoms from this.
3   Multiple factors contribute to its development.
4   Crepe bandaging can cure this.
5   Minimally invasive techniques can be effective.

Stems

A   Atherosclerosis.
B   Venous insufficiency.
C   Venous ulceration.
D   Carotid stenosis.
E   Gall stones.

Question 7. Risk factor management

Options

1 Male >45.
2 Female <50.
3 Hypertension.
4 Homocysteine metabolic abnormality.
5 Diabetes mellitus.
6 HDL/total cholesterol ratio less than 20%.
7 Total cholesterol 6.5.

Stems

A Treatment with a statin is appropriate.
B Can be modified to reduce risk of PVD.
C Is associated with an increased risk of PVD.

Question 8. Treatment

Patients presenting with stable PVD.

Options

1 Should not receive aspirin.
2 Statin therapy is too costly.
3 Should only receive medical therapy.
4 Enteric coated aspirin alone.
5 Clopidogrel as a first-line drug.
6 Aspirin, and a statin.
7 Long-acting nitrates are effective.
8 Beta-blockers may be helpful.
9 Control of hypertension.
10 Proton pump inhibitor.

Stems

A   65-year-old male with angina and claudication.
B   Amaurosis fugax in a 55-year-old.
C   Intermittent claudication with history of duodenal ulceration.
D   Abdominal aortic aneurysm, male, 5.4cm anteroposterior diameter, asymptomatic.

Question 9. Carotid anatomy

Options

1   Internal jugular vein.
2   Vagus nerve.
3   Trigeminal nerve.
4   Facial nerve.
5   Accessory nerve.
6   Hypoglossal nerve.
7   Phrenic nerve.
8   Spinal accessory nerve.
9   Ansa cervicalis (descendens hypoglossi).
10   Internal carotid artery.

Stems

A   Are almost always clearly seen and preserved in carotid surgery.
B   Is medial to the internal carotid artery.
C   Is superficial to the sternomastoid.
D   Passes inferiorly from the Hypoglossal nerve.
E   Has no branches in the neck.

Question 10. Subclavian occlusion

With reference to the following angiographic abnormality.

Options

1   Occlusion of the left subclavian artery.
2   Occlusion of inomminate artery.
3   Refilling of subclavian via retrograde flow in vertebral artery.
4   Presents with right arm claudication.
5   Dizziness, diplopia, unsteady gait.
6   Only treatable by angioplasty and stenting.
7   Left carotid subclavian bypass or transposition.

Stems

A   What statements are true?
B   What treatment options are available?
C   May cause radiofemoral delay.
D   Blood pressure measured in both arms will be equal.

Question 11. Thoracic outlet syndrome

Options

1   A patient presents with a chronically swollen upper limb.
2   Acute swelling upper limb with superficial venous distension.
3   History of discomfort along the ulnar border of the forearm for several months associated with small muscle weakness and wasting.
4   Paraesthesia at night affecting the radial three fingers.
5   Unilateral Raynauds' syndrome.
6   Blanching of the finger tips and numbness on exposure to vibration or cold.
7   Asymptomatic.

Stems

A   Axillary vein thrombosis.
B   Paget Schroetter syndrome.
C   Cervical rib.
D   Thoracic outlet syndrome.
E   Ulnar neuropathy.
F   Carpal tunnel syndrome.
G   Lymphoedema.
H   Hand arm vibration syndrome (HAVS).

Question 12. Assessment

You are the SHO in the vascular clinic and are presented with these patients. Old notes are not available. Best management requires:

Options

1   Random glucose.
2   Fasting lipids.
3   Homocysteine levels.
4   Thrombophilia screen.
5   Full blood count.
6   Urea and electrolytes.
7   Liver function tests.
8   ECG.
9   CT brain.
10   Carotid duplex ultrasound.

Stems

A   76-year-old woman with recent hemiplegic stroke.
B   Young patient <50 years acute ischaemia of leg 3 months ago.
C   Intermittent claudicant aged 65 years.
D   60-year-old man, 3/12 post-myocardial infarction complicated by peripheral embolisation.
E   95-year-old woman with single digit gangrene.

Question 13. Emergency case

You are the SHO in surgery called to the A&E department and have been given a list of patient diagnoses. Unfortunately, the A&E officer has just gone off-duty and has not listed which patient is which!

Options

1   ?Renal colic.
2   ?Urothelial malignancy.
3   ?Leaking aortic aneurysm.
4   ?Diverticular disease.
5   ?Muscular strain.
6   ?Ectopic pregnancy.

Stems

A   78-year-old man with sudden onset left-sided severe abdominal pain from loin to groin, BP120/80mmHg, pulse 90/min.
B   65-year-old woman with a 2-day history of left iliac fossa pain, colicky initially, associated with pyrexia.
C   50-year-old man 6-hour history of left-sided loin to groin pain, blood on dipstick.
D   35-year-old female, pale, clammy, BP 90/50 mmHg.

Question 14. Aortic aneurysm disease

Options

1   6cm anteroposterior aortic diameter.
2   4cm anteroposterior aortic diameter.
3   Tender AAA known to be 6cm.
4   Expansion of 0.75cm in one year.
5   Male 70 years of age, collapse with severe back pain.
6   Inflammatory 6cm AAA.

Stems

A   Annual ultrasound scan.
B   Emergency repair.
C   Repair on next elective risk.

D   Elective repair.
E   Ureteric stents should be inserted.

Question 15. Aneurysmal disease (general)

Options

1   Is only acceptable as part of a randomised control trial.
2   Only suitable if unfit for open surgery.
3   Is associated with better long-term results.
4   Is associated with reduced morbidity and mortality.
5   Never results in late rupture.
6   Popliteal aneurysm is best treated by ...

Stems

A   Open repair.
B   Endoluminal repair.
C   Axillobifemoral graft.
D   Femoropopliteal graft.

Question 16. Complications of vascular surgery

Options

1   Embolism.
2   Rupture.
3   Thrombosis.
4   Infection.
5   Myocardial infarction.
6   Pneumonia.
7   Bleeding.
8   Graft infection.
9   Aortoenteric fistula.
10   False aneurysm.
11   Deep venous thrombosis.
12   Compartment syndrome.
13   Arterial dissection.
14   Acute limb ischaemia.

Stems

A Aortic aneurysm.
B General postoperative complications.
C Popliteal aneurysm.
D Cardiac catheterisation.
E PTFE femoropopliteal bypass.

Question 17. Renal artery stenosis

Pathology/diagnosis/treatment.

Options

1 Young hypertensive patient, without family history.
2 Smoker.
3 Responds well to angioplasty.
4 Deteriorating renal function.
5 Normal renal function.
6 Resistant hypertension.
7 Older patients.
8 Usually affects women.
9 Flash pulmonary oedema.
10 Minimal proteinuria.
11 No prospect of recovery with intervention.

Stems

A Fibromuscular dysplasia.
B Atherosclerotic renal artery stenosis.
C Ostial renal artery stenosis.
D Renal size <8cm bilaterally (in adults).

Question 18. Critical ischaemia

Options

1 Ulceration secondary to minimal pressure or adjacent toes.
2 Pain in the foot on standing upright.
3 Sensation of walking on pebbles.
4 Nocturnal pain relieved by dependency.
5 Palpable foot pulses.
6 ABPI >1.5.
7 Ankle pressure <50mmHg.
8 Reduced sensation in stocking distribution.

Stems

A Diabetic with significant neurovascular disease.
B Spinal stenosis.
C Critical limb ischaemia.
D Indication for angiography.
E Indication for intervention.

Question 19. Sutures, embolectomy and grafts

Match wherever possible the vessel to the surgical options.

Options

1 5Fr Fogarty catheter.
2 3/0 prolene.
3 5/0 Goretex (PTFE).
4 3/0 silk.
5 3Fr Foley catheter.
6 2Fr Fogarty catheter.
7 20mm Dacron graft.
8 6mm PTFE graft with Miller cuff.
9 8mm PTFE graft.
10 4/0 prolene.
11 6/0 prolene.
12 7/0 prolene.

Stems

A   Iliac artery.
B   Aorta.
C   Brachial artery.
D   Above knee popliteal artery.
E   Posterior tibial artery.
F   Below knee popliteal artery.

Question 20. Leg ulcers

Options

1   Atypical non-healing ulcer.
2   Rolled edge in chronic ulcer (many years).
3   Gaiter area of leg, with brown staining of the skin.
4   Over base of 5th metatarsal or head of first metatarsal.
5   Deformed joints of foot with punched out ulcer.
6   Lateral malleolus, or heel.
7   Multiple small superficial ulcers, with haemorrhagic rash.

Stems

A   Venous ulcer.
B   Arterial ulcer.
C   Malignant ulcer.
D   Neuropathic ulcer.
E   Vasculitic.

Question 21. The swollen leg

Swelling of the lower limb.

Options

1 Acute onset unilateral swollen leg.
2 Swollen legs from birth.
3 Pitting oedema of both lower limbs.
4 Clinical diagnosis possible from history and clinical findings.
5 MRI shows a typical 'honeycomb' appearance of the soft tissues.
6 Hyperkeratosis (warty appearance of the skin).
7 Both legs affected.
8 Feet not affected.

Stems

A Inferior vena cava obstruction.
B Congestive cardiac failure.
C Deep vein thrombosis.
D Lymphoedema praecox.
E Congenital lymphoedema.
F Pelvic malignancy.
G Lipoedema.

Answer 1   A2 & 7, B3, 8,10 &12, C3, 4, 6, 8 &10, D11,12 & 13, E none

Differential diagnosis of leg pain requires a careful detailed history. Often the patient is elderly and has more than one pathology to account for their symptoms. Often the diagnosis is not made until results of ABPI, exercise ABPI, x-ray of hip and knee are available.

Answer 2   A3, B2 & 3, C1, 2, 3, 4, 5 & 6, D none

Attempting to assess the level of vascular occlusion can be of help and combined with careful clinical examination can often determine the level of the arterial occlusion. This can help with planning of further investigation and management.

Answer 3   A4,11 & 13, B1, 5, 11, 13 & (7), C1, 4, 7, 8, 11 & (12), D4 & 13, E none

It is good practice to review notes in the outpatients to review history, ensure correct patient, diagnosis and results of previous investigations. This prevents duplication of investigations, waste and overlooking positive results. All conditions can be affected by thrombocytosis. Atherosclerosis in young people can be associated with hyperhomocysteinaemia, an abnormality of folate metabolism.

In the absence of an aortic aneurysm screening programme, opportunistic screening of all patients with cerebrovascular, cardiac or peripheral vascular disease is advisable.

The Asymptomatic Carotid Surgery Trial results suggest that patients with carotid stenoses >70% in with a life expectancy of more than 3 years benefit from carotid endarterectomy. Carotid bruits should now be taken seriously; however, a tight stenosis of 95% or more may not give a bruit!

Answer 4   A2, 3 & 4, B5 & 6, C1 & 7, D2 & 3, E none, F8

The typical visual disturbance from a carotid stenosis is ipsilateral transient loss of vision (amaurosis fugax). It can result in permanent field loss or blindness in the affected eye. If the embolus lodges more posteriorly, field loss can occur in both eyes. This can cause quadrantic or homonomous hemianopias.

In right-handed people the speech centre is usually located in the contralateral hemisphere to the dominant hand, i.e. in right-handed people it is usually in the left hemisphere (Stem 2).

Answer 5   A1 & (5), B1, (3 & 5), C1 & 2, D1, 3 & 5, E1, 3 & 5, F1

The modern diagnosis of vascular disease utilises several modalities and is becoming less invasive. Magnetic resonance techniques exclude radiation exposure, and are providing increasing definition approaching that of intra-arterial digital subtraction angiography. The basic principle of investigation restricts invasive diagnostic techniques for those in whom intervention (open or endovascular) is contemplated. The information obtained non-invasively is likely to allow for planned percutaneous intervention rather then a diagnostic invasive test followed by a subsequent percutaneous procedure.

Answer 6   A1, 3 & 5, B2 & 5, C(5), D5, E5

Answer 7   A7, B4, 5 & 7, C1, 3, 4, 5 & 7

Answer 8   A6, 7 & 8, B6 & 9 (this patient should also undergo
                  urgent Duplex ultrasound of the carotid vessels), C6,10
                  (4, 5 may also be used in combination with 10), D3 & 9

Patients should receive optimal therapy for all treatable risk factors, regardless of apparent cost. Comorbidities eg. peptic ulceration needs careful consideration. Treatment with a proton pump inhibitor (PPI) can allow safer aspirin administration. The use of cardioselective betablockers is not thought to adversely affect claudication and may have a protective effect against myocardial infarction. Control of hypertension is exceptionally important in stroke prevention, and also has a role in prevention of aneurysm enlargement.

Answer 9 A1, 2 & 4, B none, C5, D9, E10

The anatomy of the carotid sheath is essential to the vascular surgeon carrying out carotid surgery.

Answer 10 A1, 3 & 5, B7, C none, D1

Subclavian occlusion is often asymptomatic but may present with symptoms associated with decreased posterior brain circulation eg. diplopia, dizziness, unsteady gait, inco-ordination. Arm claudication may occur. The collateral supply to the upper limb is considerable; the proximal subclavian artery is used by paediatric cardiothoracic surgeons to patch coarctation of the aorta without any problems to the left arm.

Answer 11 A1 & 2, B2, C1, 2, 3 & 7, D1, 2, 3, 4 & 5, E3, F4, G1, H6

HAVS was previously known as hand arm vibration syndrome. Paget Scroetter syndrome is axillary vein thrombosis secondary to obstruction to the thoracic outlet by a band of tissue or cervical rib. Thoracic Outlet Syndrome most frequently presents with neurological symptoms causing brachialgia and unilateral Raynauds. It can also present with venous obstruction or thrombosis. Arterial thoracic outlet is least common but can present with distal embolisation from local arterial trauma, or ischaemia due to occlusion of the subclavian artery or stenosis with post-stenotic dilatation with embolisation or aneurysm formation.

Answer 12 A1, 2, 5, 8, 9 & 10, B1, 2, 3, 4 & 8, C1, 2 & 5, D1, 2, 5 & 8, E5

PVD is a reflection of the vascular system as a whole. Mortality is usually cardiac in origin and morbidity from stroke, or limb loss is considerable. Risk factors need assessment and modulation to avoid life-threatening complications. Comorbidity for example from undiagnosed diabetes mellitus is common. Treatable conditions can modify the outcome for the patient.

It is important to note and modulate risk factors; however, at the age of 95 it is likely that the only risk factor to be modified would be platelet stabilisation with aspirin (in the absence of a history of peptic ulceration).

Answer 13   A3, B4, C1 & 2, (3), D6

Elderly male patients with undiagnosed abdominal pain and hypotension, or first episode of renal colic need to be treated as a leaking abdominal aortic aneurysm. Prompt diagnosis and surgical intervention can reduce in-hospital mortality to as low as 20% in some centres. Although some surgeons will insist on imaging prior to intervention, it is the authors' belief that in the presence of the above triad of advanced age, collapse and backpain, that urgent surgery is the definitive diagnostic and therapeutic procedure! Ultrasound is not sensitive or specific enough to exclude a leaking AAA. The delay obtaining a CT scan can result in the patient's death in the CT scanner (the euphemistic 'doughnut of death').

Answer 14   A2, B5, C3, D1, E none

The small aneurysm trial has demonstrated that the risk of surgery exceeds the benefit in aneurysms <5.5cm. Aneurysm repair is associated with roughly 8-9% risk of morbidity including a mortality of up to 5%. If the patient is otherwise fit and well, elective mortality should be in the order of 2%. If the aneurysm expands rapidly i.e. >1cm in one year, or if it is symptomatic, i.e. painful or tender, then surgery is indicated. Inflammatory aneurysms are frequently associated with ureteric obstruction and renal compromise. They are often difficult to identify at surgery; stenting can improve renal function and help identify and therefore reduce injury to the ureter.

Answer 15   A3, B4, C none, D6

Endoluminal repair is currently being evaluated by several national and international trials, (eg. EVAR and EVAR2). The long-term outcome of these procedures is awaited. The technology is progressing and therefore, results of early trials are likely to be surpassed by newer devices.

74

EMQs for surgery

Answer 16 A1, 2, 3, 4 & 7, B1, 2, 3, 4, 5, 6, 7, 8, 10, 11, 12, C1, 2, 3, 4, 5, 7, (8, 10), 11,12 & 14, D1, 5, 7, 10, 13 & 14, E3, 4, 7 & 8

It is important to have a high index of suspicion for complications of vascular surgery and also those of the investigations carried out in the diagnosis and pre-operative investigation of the arteriopath. These are high-risk patients undergoing high-risk procedures.

Answer 17 A1, 3, 5, 6, 8, 9 &10, B2, (3), 4, 6, 7, 9 &10, C4, 6, 9 & 10, D11

Renal artery stenosis remains difficult to treat. Decisions are mainly made according to response to medical therapy, and potential for reducing end organ damage and preserving renal function. Revascularisation is nearly always by interventional radiology. Surgery is reserved for resistant or failed radiological procedures.

Answer 18 A1, 3, 4, 6, (7) & 8, B5, C1, 4 & 7, D1 & 4, E1, 4 & 7

Critical ischaemia requires intervention if tissue loss (digit or limb) is to be avoided. ABPI can be inaccurate in patients with diabetes, due to medial calcification; however, if the pressure is low this is significant in itself. Angiography should only be carried out if considering intervention. ABPI <0.5, or an absolute pressure <50mmHg, presence of ulceration, or gangrene is an effective working definition for critical ischaemia.

Answer 19 A1 &10, B1, 2, 7 & (10)*, C11, D3, 9 & 11, E6,11 &12, F8 & 11

The choice of suture and graft material is complex. If prosthetic grafts are used in the leg, especially in the below knee segment, they have a lower long-term patency rate despite the use of adjuncts such as the Miller cuff, Taylor patch, Karacagil patch or Mary's boot. It was previously thought that PTFE grafts used above the knee had as good an outcome as vein grafts. Recent evidence has shown this to be untrue. *If the aorta is very friable and there is suture line bleeding, use of a more delicate suture can be most effective.

Answer 20   A3, B4 & 6, C1 & 2, D4 & 5, E7

Answer 21   A3, 4 & 7, B3 & 7, C1, D4, 5, 6 & 7, E2, 3, 4, 5, 6 & 7, F1, G7 & 8

Chapter 5

Venous disease

Alun H Davies, MA DM FRCS
Reader in Surgery and Consultant Surgeon,
Imperial College School of Medicine, Charing Cross Hospital, London, UK
Louis J Fligelstone, MB BCh FRCS (Eng) FRCS (Gen)
Consultant Surgeon, Morriston Hospital, Swansea, UK

For all questions each option may be used once, more than once or not at all.

Question 1. Varicose veins

Options

1   Deep vein thrombosis.
2   Superficial vein thrombosis.
3   Long saphenous vein incompetence.
4   Short saphenous vein incompetence.
5   Perforator incompetence.

Stems

A   Is best managed by a NSAID.
B   Compression hosiery should always be used in this condition.
C   Can only be diagnosed by ascending venography.
D   May revert to competence following venous surgery.
E   Can be associated with malignancy.

Question 2. Ulcer

Options

1   Venous ulcer.
2   Squamous cell carcinoma.
3   Traumatic ulcers.
4   Arterial ulceration.
5   Fasciotomy scars.

Stems

A   Rheumatoid factor is known to be associated with poor healing.
B   Diabetes is an independent factor associated with healing.
C   Healing rate is improved by long saphenous vein surgery.
D   Can be appropriately treated by an Unna boot.

Question 3. Lower limb disease

Options

1   Deep vein thrombosis.
2   Erythema abignea.
3   Phlegmasia caerulea dolens.
4   Necrobiosis lipodica.

Stems

A   Is associated with diabetes mellitus.
B   Can be prevented by subcutaneous heparin.
C   Can be treated by thrombolysis.

Question 4. Venous thrombosis

Options

1   Non-fatal pulmonary embolism.
2   Fatal pulmonary embolism.
3   Iliac vein thrombosis.
4   Femoral vein thrombosis.
5   Calf vein thrombosis.

Stems

A   Is reduced by the use of subcutaneous heparin.
B   Is reduced by the use of TEDS.
C   Is associated with obesity.
D   Is associated with breast malignancy.

Question 5. Diagnosis

Which of the following is the most likely diagnosis in the following clinical scenario?

Options

1   Pulmonary embolism.
2   Deep vein thrombosis.
3   Myocardial infarction.
4   Pneumonia.

Stems

A   A 72-year-old patient 6 days post-surgery complains of 2 hours of chest pain and cough. His PaO_2 is 8.3kPa and $PaCo_2$ of 3.5kPa.
B   57-year-old man 24 hours post-nephrectomy collapses. His ECG shows left ventricular strain.
C   Is the commonest cause of death following a fractured neck of femur.

Question 6. Upper limb disease

Options

1 Raynaud's Syndrome.
2 Cervical rib.
3 Buerger's disease.
4 Scleroderma.
5 SLE.

Stems

A Is often associated with cold exposure.
B Normally presents with lower limb symptoms.
C Should be routinely excised to prophylatically prevent upper limb symptoms.
D Throrascopic sympathectomy may be used in the treatment of this condition.

Question 7. Associations with venous disease

Options

1 Long saphenous vein incompetence.
2 Pregnancy.
3 Smoking.
4 Protein C deficiency.
5 Fractured neck of femur.

Stems

A Is associated with a 10-fold increased risk of DVT.
B Occurs in up to 10% of women under the age of 20.

Question 8. Investigation

Which is the most appropriate investigation in the following scenarios?

Options

1 CT angiography.
2 Lower limb duplex.
3 V/Q scan.
4 Chest x-ray.
5 D-dimer.

Stems

A A 41-year-old presents with haemoptysis following surgery. What is the definitive diagnostic test for a PE?

B Is the most sensitive test to confirm an early diagnosis of deep vein thrombosis.

Question 9. Vein type

Options

1 Long saphenous vein.
2 Short saphenous vein.
3 Cephalic vein.
4 Basilic vein.
5 Internal jugular vein.

Stems

A Surgical removal of this vein can be associated with numbness on the calf.

B Mobilization of this vein can result in damage to the medial cutaneous nerve.

C Incompetent perforators can return to competence after removal of this vein.

D This vein is often used as a transposition graft in the creation of an AV fistula.

Question 10. Nerve or vein damage

Options

1   Damage to the common peroneal nerve.
2   Damage to the femoral nerve.
3   Division and ligation of the popliteal vein.
4   Division and damage to the superficial femoral vein.
5   Damage to the sciatic nerve.

Stems

A   A 52-year-old lady complains of inability to extend the ankle following varicose vein surgery.
B   A 42-year-old female develops a swollen, painful leg 8 hours after surgery to the short saphenous vein.
C   A 65-year-old complains of severe pain and swelling in the leg while in recovery following a femoropopliteal bypass.

Question 11. Treatment

Which is the most appropriate treatment option in the following scenarios?

Options

1   Nifedipine.
2   Iloprost.
3   Endoscopic thorascopic sympathectomy.
4   Bendrofluazide.
5   Trental.

Stems

A   A 52-year-old lady presents with recent onset Raynaud's disease. What is the first line pharmacological treatment?
B   Gustatory sweating is associated with this treatment.
C   A 68-year-old presents to the pre-admission clinic prior to her varicose vein treatment. Her serum K+ comes back at 3.3mMol/L. Which medication would you stop?
D   Administration of this/these medications to a patient with a vasospastic disorder is associated with headache.

Question 12. Investigation

Which single investigation would give you the most reliable confirmation of diagnosis?

Options

1   Duplex.
2   Venography.
3   Lymphangiography.
4   CT scan.
5   Arteriography.

Stems

A   Popliteal entrapment.
B   Deep vein incompetence.
C   Milroy's disease.
D   Paget Schroetter Syndrome.

Question 13. Differential diagnosis

Options

1   Popliteal entrapment.
2   Deep vein thrombosis.
3   Compartment syndrome.
4   Acute arterial occlusion.
5   Lymphoedema.

Stems

A   A 32-year-old professional soccer player complains of pain in the calf for 2 months on walking 200yds.
B   A 63-year-old lady complains of pain in the calf 12 hours after a coronary angiogram.
C   5 hours following a femoral embolectomy, the patient complains of severe pain and swelling of the calf and it is noted that his urine output has tailed off to less than 10mls per hour.

Question 14. Associations

Options

1   Homocystinemia.
2   Rheumatoid factor.
3   Elevated CRP.
4   Anaemia.
5   Uraemia.

Stems

A   Venous disease is more common in patients with this condition.
B   Factors that are associated with poor healing of gaiter leg ulcers.

Question 15. Complications of venous surgery

Options

1   Recurrence.
2   Sciatic nerve damage.
3   Bruising in thigh.
4   Numbness in the skin.
5   Foot drop.
6   Deep vein thrombosis.

Stems

A   Long saphenous vein surgery.
B   Short saphenous vein surgery.
C   Avulsion of the anterior thigh vein.
D   Cephalic vein harvest.

Question 16. Symptoms and signs

Which symptoms and signs are the most likely to be associated with:

Options

1 Heaviness.
2 Aching.
3 Pigmentation.
4 Swelling.
5 Leg ulceration.
6 Rest pain.
7 Claudication.
8 Redness/inflammation on leg.

Stems

A Long saphenous vein incompetence.
B Short saphenous vein incompetence.
C Superficial femoral vein occlusion.
D Popliteal vein occlusion.
E Superficial vein thrombosis.

| Answer 1 | A2, B1, C none, D5, E1 & 2 |

| Answer 2 | A1, B4 & 3, C1, D1 |

| Answer 3 | A4, B1, C1 & 3 |

| Answer 4 | A1, 3, 4 & 5, B1, 3, 4 & 5, C1 - 5, D1 - 5 |

| Answer 5 | A1, B1, C4 |

| Answer 6 | A1, B3, C none, D1, 3, 4 & 5 |

| Answer 7 | A2, B1 |

| Answer 8 | A1, B2 |

| Answer 9 | A2, B4, C1, D4 |

| Answer 10 | A1 & 5, B3, C4 |

| Answer 11 | A1, B3, C4, D1 & 2 |

| Answer 12 | A4, B2, C3, D2 |

Duplex in many cases may be the first-line investigation. However, as in popliteal entrapment, CT angiography is probably regarded as the gold standard (as is MRI).

| Answer 13 | A1, B4, C3 |

| Answer 14 | A1, B1, 2, 4 & 5 |

Answer 15   A1, 3, 4 & 6, B1, 2, 4, 5 & 6, C1, 3, 4 & 6, D4 & 6

Answer 16   A1, 2, 3, 4 & 5
B1, 2, 3, 4 & 5
C1, 2, 3, 4, 5 & 7, symptoms of claudication are rare
D1, 2, 3, 4, 5 & 7, symptoms of claudication are rare
E1, 2, 4 & 8

Symptoms of superficial and venous disease can be very difficult to
exactly define.

Chapter 6

Cardiothoracic surgery

Afzal Zaidi, MA MB BChir FRCS (C-Th)
Consultant Cardiothoracic Surgeon, Morriston Hospital, Swansea, UK
Heyman Luckraz, MB BS FRCS
Specialist Registrar, Cardiothoracic Surgery, Morriston Hospital, Swansea, UK

For all questions each option may be used once, more than once or not at all.

Question 1. The most common surgical approach

Options

1   Median sternotomy.
2   Right posterolateral thoracotomy.
3   Left posterolateral thoracotomy.
4   Video-assisted thoracoscopy.
5   Mediastinoscopy.

Stems

A   Left upper lobectomy for carcinoma.
B   Biopsy of paratracheal lymph nodes.
C   Aortic valve replacement.
D   Pleural biopsy.
E   Repair of aortic transection.

Question 2. Anatomy of the coronary tree

Options

1   Right coronary artery.
2   Left main stem.
3   Left anterior descending artery.
4   Obtuse marginal artery.
5   Posterior descending artery.

Stems

A   Most commonly supplies the sino-atrial node.
B   Is most commonly dominant.
C   The main supply for the interventricular septum.
D   Severe stenosis is a definite indication for coronary bypass surgery.
E   Is a branch of the circumflex artery.

Question 3. Pre-operative investigations of cardiac disease

Options

1   Resting electrocardiogram.
2   Exercise electrocardiogram.
3   Transthoracic echocardiography.
4   Transoesophageal echocardiography.
5   Coronary angiography.

Stems

A   May be normal in a patient with significant coronary artery disease.
B   Is used as a screening test in patients with angina.
C   Gives the best assessment of the mitral valve.
D   Should be performed to exclude coronary artery disease in a 50-year-old man awaiting aortic valve replacement.
E   Is routinely used to assess left ventricular function.

Question 4. Cardiac surgery

Options

1   Noradrenaline.
2   Dopamine.
3   Cardioplegia.
4   Heparin.
5   Protamine.

Stems

A   Must be given prior to initiating cardiopulmonary bypass.
B   Is used to protect the myocardium.
C   May cause profound hypotension on administration.
D   Is commonly used in septic shock.
E   Can be given orally.

Question 5. Cardiac disease

Options

1   Ischaemic heart disease.
2   Aortic stenosis.
3   Aortic regurgitation.
4   Mitral regurgitation.
5   Mitral stenosis.

Stems

A   Classically presents with effort syncope.
B   Is only caused by rheumatic fever.
C   Causes left ventricular hypertrophy.
D   Can complicate a myocardial infarction.
E   Can occur in Marfan's syndrome.

Question 6. Clinical features of cardiac disease

Options

1 Ischaemic heart disease.
2 Aortic stenosis.
3 Aortic regurgitation.
4 Mitral regurgitation.
5 Mitral stenosis.

Stems

A Is associated with a malar flush.
B Is associated with a collapsing pulse.
C Severe disease may be asymptomatic.
D Can cause a pan-systolic murmur at the apex.
E Is associated with a tapping apex beat.

Question 7. Valves

Options

1 Bioprosthetic valve.
2 Mechanical valve.
3 Homograft.
4 Valve repair.
5 Heart transplantation.

Stems

A Is the best option for a 75-year-old patient with severe aortic stenosis.
B Needs lifelong anticoagulation.
C Is the best option for a 30-year-old woman with severe mitral regurgitation.
D Is ideal for a patient with aortic root abscess.
E Has the longest durability.

Question 8. Conduits for coronary artery bypass surgery

Options

1   Radial artery.
2   Left internal mammary artery.
3   Long saphenous vein.
4   Right internal mammary artery.
5   PTFE graft.

Stems

A   Has been proven to improve survival and has a better patency rate when grafted to the left anterior descending artery.
B   Has a 40% attrition rate at 10 years.
C   Suitability should be assessed by the Allen's test.
D   Has the poorest short-term patency.
E   Should be avoided in an obese diabetic patient.

Question 9. Thoracic anatomy

Options

1   Phrenic nerve.
2   Vagus nerve.
3   Main bronchus.
4   Pulmonary artery.
5   Pulmonary vein.

Stems

A   Is the most posterior hilar structure.
B   Lies on the lateral surface of the superior vena cava.
C   Runs anterior to the hilum.
D   Trauma may lead to a fatal air embolism.
E   Carries deoxygenated blood.

Question 10. Investigations for thoracic disease

Options

1   Chest radiograph.
2   Helical computed tomography.
3   Positron emission tomography scan.
4   Pulmonary function test.
5   Mediastinoscopy.

Stems

A   Is the gold standard for assessment of the mediastinal lymph nodes in lung cancer.
B   Is the first-line investigation in a 68-year-old smoker with haemoptysis.
C   Is the investigation of choice for diagnosing pulmonary embolism.
D   A 40-year-old female is found to have a solitary nodule on a routine chest radiograph. CT scan shows a smooth 1.5cm nodule with no lymphadenopahy. What should be the next investigation?
E   Is essential to assess fitness for lung resection.

Question 11. Pulmonary pathology

Options

1   Adenocarcinoma.
2   Squamous cell carcinoma.
3   Small cell carcinoma.
4   Large cell carcinoma.
5   Pulmonary metastasis from previously excised sarcoma.

Stems

A   Is not managed surgically.
B   Metastasises late.
C   Has the poorest prognosis.
D   May be associated with finger clubbing.
E   Is most radiosensitive.

Question 12. What would be the best first-line treatment?

Options

1   Chest radiograph.
2   Intercostal drain insertion.
3   Arterial blood gas analysis.
4   Endotracheal intubation.
5   Thoracotomy.

Stems

A   A 30-year-old motorcyclist with a flail chest (fractured ribs 2-8) who is haemodynamically stable and has a PCO_2 of 9KPa.
B   A 20-year-old man presents with two stab wound injuries to the left chest, lateral to the nipple. He was haemodynamically stable but a chest radiograph shows a pleural collection.
C   A 25-year-old motor cyclist crashes in a lamppost at 50 Mph. She is haemodynamically stable but a chest radiograph shows a widened mediastinum, fractured left clavicle and first rib, apical shadow with possible pleural collection.

Question 13. Lung function test

Options

1   FEV1.
2   FVC.
3   FEV1/FVC.
4   PEFR.
5   TV.

Stems

A   The volume of air breathed in at rest.
B   The predicted postoperative value determines the extent of lung resection that a patient could tolerate.
C   May be normal in restrictive lung disease.
D   Is the simplest to measure as an outpatient.
E   Can be used to diagnose pulmonary embolism.

Question 14. Complications of lung resection

Options

1   Broncho-pleural fistula.
2   Empyema.
3   Atelectasis.
4   Bleeding.
5   Acute lung injury.

Stems

A   May be prevented by adequate analgesia and physiotherapy.
B   May result from prolonged intercostal drainage for air leak.
C   Is more common after pneumonectomy on the right than on the left.
D   May be due to systemic inflammatory response syndrome.
E   Should be treated by prompt intercostal drainage.

Question 15. Pleural collection

Options

1   Pneumothorax.
2   Haemothorax.
3   Chylothorax.
4   Pleural effusion.
5   Empyema.

Stems

A   Most likely to develop in a patient with mesothelioma.
B   May lead to profound hypoalbuminaemia.
C   May be caused by hypoalbuminaemia.
D   Typically occurs in tall, thin young adults.
E   May be associated with leucocytosis on microscopy.

Question 16. These percentages represent

Options

1 Less than 5%.
2 Greater than 50%.
3 Greater than 90%.
4 Around 20%.
5 5-10%.

Stems

A The percentage of resectable lung cancer.
B Is the 5-year survival after resection of stage I lung cancer.
C Is the quoted surgical mortality to a fit patient undergoing lung lobar resection.
D Represents the incidence of broncho-pleural fistula post-lung resection.
E Is the mortality rate after pneumonectomy.

Question 17. Congenital heart disease

Options

1 Atrial septal defect
2 Ventricular septal defect
3 Tetralogy of Fallot
4 Patent ductus arteriosus
5 Coarctation of the aorta

Stems

A Causes cyanosis in childhood.
B Is associated with rib notching on the chest radiograph.
C Is associated with a continuous machinery murmur.
D May be multiple.
E May be the cause of a paradoxical embolus in a previously fit 20-year-old.

Question 18. Associated complications of cardiac surgery

Options

1   Diabetes mellitus.
2   Obesity.
3   Chronic obstructive pulmonary disease.
4   Peripheral vascular disease.
5   Hypokalaemia.

Stems

A   Wound infection.
B   Non-infected sternal dehiscence.
C   Atrial fibrillation (AF).
D   Stroke.
E   Pneumothorax.

Question 19. Management of ischaemic heart disease

Options

1   Coronary bypass surgery.
2   Percutaneous coronary intervention.
3   Medical therapy.
4   Transmyocardial laser revascularisation.
5   Transplantation.

Stems

A   Patient with stable angina and 90% left main stem stenosis.
B   Patient with chest pain and a normal exercise test electrocardiogram (12 minutes of Bruce protocol).
C   50-year-old man with severe angina and isolated discrete single vessel stenosis and good left ventricular function.
D   A 42-year-old man with multiple previous MIs, previous CABG, poor left ventricular function (EF of 10%), no revascularisable myocardium on perfusion scan, and no graftable vessels on angiography.
E   Patient with class III angina, severe three vessel disease, with moderate left ventricular function.

Question 20. Cardiological investigation

Options

1   P wave.
2   Dichrotic notch.
3   QRS complex.
4   T wave.
5   A wave.

Stems

A   Occurs at the onset of diastole.
B   Indicates activation through the His-Purkinje system.
C   Ventricular repolarisation.
D   May be peaked in pulmonary hypertension.
E   May be peaked in hyperkalaemia.

Question 21. Heart murmurs

Options

1   Ejection systolic murmur.
2   Pan-systolic murmur.
3   Early diastolic murmur.
4   Mid diastolic murmur.
5   Continuous machinery murmur.

Stems

A   Mitral stenosis.
B   Ventricular septal defect.
C   Ruptured sinus of Valsalva aneurysm.
D   Aortic stenosis.
E   Aortic regurgitation.

Question 22. Early complications of cardiac surgery

Options

1   Hypovolaemia.
2   Cardiac tamponade.
3   Mesenteric ischaemia.
4   Left ventricular failure.
5   Pulmonary embolism.

Stems

A   A 65-year-old ventilated male arteriopathic patient develops a worsening acidosis and leucocytosis following cardiac surgery.
B   Decreased JVP, decreased blood pressure, decreased urine output, normal pH.
C   Increased JVP, decreased blood pressure, decreased urine output, decreased pH.
D   Is best treated with intra-aortic balloon pump.
E   Causes profound hypoxia.

Question 23. Blood tests

Options

1   Cholesterol levels.
2   Troponin.
3   VDRL.
4   Creatinine.
5   APTT.

Stems

A   Should be checked in a patient with a dilated aortic root.
B   Should be monitored in a patient on an ACE inhibitor.
C   Is a marker of myocardial cell damage.
D   Describes the extrinsic coagulation pathway.
E   Is an important part of secondary prevention for ischaemic heart disease.

Question 24. Complications of cardiac surgery

Options

1   Less than 5%.
2   5-10%.
3   20-40%.
4   50-60%.
5   Greater than 80%.

Stems

A   Incidence of atrial fibrillation after CABG.
B   Incidence of stroke after CABG.
C   Is the mortality after elective CABG.
D   Represents the patency rate of saphenous vein grafts at 10 years.
E   Represents the patency rate of LIMA at 10 years.

Question 25. Intracardiac disease

Options

1   Atrial septal defect.
2   Ventricular septal defect (VSD).
3   Mitral regurgitation.
4   Aortic regurgitation.
5   Mitral stenosis.

Stems

A   May be caused by acute MI.
B   May be caused by aortic dissection.
C   May be caused by endocarditis.
D   An Intra-Aortic Balloon Pump (IABP) is an absolute contraindication.
E   Is only caused by rheumatic fever.

Answer 1   A3, B5 (B4), C1, D4, E3

Median sternotomy is the incision of choice for access to the heart and proximal great vessels, as well as the anterior mediastinum eg. thymectomy. Posterolateral thoracotomy is the incision of choice for lung resections, oesophageal surgery and surgery of the descending thoracic aorta (left). Paratracheal lymph nodes are biopsied via a mediastinoscope in the staging of lung cancer. Video-assisted thoracoscopy ('VATS') is commonly used for lung and pleural biopsies, as well as pleurodesis for pneumothorax.

Answer 2   A1, B1, C3, D2, E4

The dominant coronary artery is defined as the one which gives rise to the posterior descending artery and is usually the right coronary artery (75%). 15% are left dominant and 10% have a balanced circulation - 'co-dominant'.

Three landmark studies in the 1970s defined the prognostic benefit for coronary artery bypass surgery over medical therapy for two groups of patients: a) patients with left mainstem stenosis; and b) patients with three vessel disease with left ventricular impairment.

Whilst some patients in group (b) could now be treated with percutaneous intervention (angioplasty/stenting), patients with left main disease should undergo CABG.

Answer 3   A1 (A3, A4), B2, C4, D5, E3

Answer 4   A4, B3, C5, D1, E none

Prior to commencing cardiopulmonary bypass the patient must be fully anticoagulated with heparin. This is reversed with protamine at the end of the procedure. Protamine must be given slowly as it may cause profound hypotension. Septic patients usually have a low systemic vascular resistance, and are thus treated (on ITU) with noradrenaline - a vasoconstrictor (alpha 1 agonist).

Answer 5   A2, B5, C2, D4, E3

Answer 6   A5, B3, C1, D4, E5

Answer 7   A1, B2, C4, D3, E2

There is no such thing as a perfect prosthetic valve; all types have advantages and disadvantages. Mechanical valves last the equivalent of 150 years when tested on the bench (!) - but the patient must take warfarin for life. The risks of warfarin increase with age, particularly over 70 years. Most surgeons therefore implant bioprostheses (tissue valves) in the over 70 age group. Modern bioprostheses last in excess of 15 years in the aortic position.

The mitral valve may be suitable for repair. This is preferable to replacement as left ventricular function is better maintained, and if the patient is in sinus rhythm, warfarin may be avoided.

Homografts are harvested from human cadavers and are thus in short supply. Homograft valve replacements are technically more demanding to perform, but being of natural tissue are more resistant to infection and are thus a good choice for complex endocarditis.

Answer 8   A2, B3, C1, D5, E4

The left internal mammary graft to the LAD is the gold standard with 15-year patency rates in excess of 95%. The next most common conduit used is long saphenous vein which shows attrition down to 60% patency at 10 years. There is a trend to use more arterial grafts in younger patients. Bilateral internal mammary arteries may be used, but should probably be avoided in obesity, diabetes and COPD to avoid sternal dehiscence. The radial artery has similar patency to saphenous vein at 7 years, but is likely to be better at 10 and 15 years (results awaited).

Artificial grafts eg. PTFE should be avoided.

EMQs for surgery

Answer 9   A3, B1, C1, D5, E4

Answer 10   A5, B1, C2, D3, E4

Positron emission tomography is useful in diagnosing or excluding malignancy in the solitary pulmonary nodule. However, there are false positives (eg. TB) and false negatives (bronchoalveolar carcinoma) associated with this investigation.

Answer 11   A3, B2, C3, D1, 2 & 4, E2

Non-small cell carcinoma is treated surgically if in an early stage (stage I, II and IIIa). Small cell carcinoma metastasises early and is treated with chemotherapy.

Answer 12   A4, B2, C5

A   The patient has acute respiratory failure and requires urgent intubation.

B   90% of stab wounds to the chest can be managed with chest drain insertion alone.

C   The patient has an aortic transection. This should be confirmed on a CT scan.

Answer 13   A5, B1, C3, D4, E none

The investigation of choice for pulmonary embolism is spiral CT scanning.

Answer 14   A3, B2, C1, D5, E1, 2 & 4

Answer 15   A4, B3, C4, D1, E3 & 5

Answer 16   A4, B2, C1, D1, E5

In the UK, the mortality for lobectomy for carcinoma is 2.5% whilst that for pneumonectomy is 7-8% (considerably higher than the majority of cardiac surgical procedures performed in the UK).

Answer 17   A3, B5, C4, D2, E1

B   Due to large collaterals via the intercostal arteries.
E   Echocardiography is mandatory in any young patient suffering a stroke or TIA.

Answer 18   A1, 2 & 4, B2 & 3, C5, D4, E3

A   Diabetes increases the risk of wound infections in any setting. Obesity increases the risk of sternal wound complications and peripheral vascular disease increases the risk of leg (vein harvest site) wound infections.
C   25% of CABG operations are complicated by postoperative AF. Hypokalaemia predisposes to AF.
D   Peripheral vascular disease is associated with carotid and ascending aortic disease.

Answer 19   A1, B3, C2, D5, E1

Answer 20   A2 & 4, B3, C4, D1, E4

Answer 21   A4, B2, C5, D1, E3

C   May rupture into the right atrium causing a continuous left to right shunt throughout the cardiac cycle.

Answer 22   A3, B1, C2 (C4, C5), D4, E5

Answer 23   A3, B4, C2, D none, E1

Answer 24   A3, B1, C1, D4, E5

Answer 25   A2 & 3, B4, C3 & 4, D4, E5

A   Post infarct mitral regurgitation (ruptured papillary muscle) and post infarction VSD are two complications of an acute MI which require urgent surgical intervention. A new murmur in the first few days after MI may herald one of these two complications.

D   An IABP requires a competent aortic valve to function (diastolic augmentation).

Chapter 7
Breast disease

Bilal A Al-Sarireh, MRCS (Ed) PhD (Eng)
Specialist Registrar, General Surgery, Morriston Hospital, Swansea, UK
Mike Chare, MA BM BCh FRCS
Consultant Breast & General Surgeon, Morriston Hospital, Swansea, UK

For all questions each option may be used once, more than once or not at all.

Question 1. Relative risk for developing breast carcinoma

Options

1   No increased risk.
2   Slight increased risk (1.1 to 2 times).
3   Moderate increased risk (2.1 to 4 times).
4   High risk (>4 times).

Stems

A   Lobular carcinoma *in situ*.
B   Duct ectasia.
C   Fibroadenoma.
D   Atypical ductal hyperplasia.
E   Cysts.

Question 2. Relative risk for developing invasive breast carcinoma

Options

1 No increased risk.
2 Slight increased risk (1.1 to 2 times).
3 Moderate increased risk (2.1 to 4 times).
4 High risk (>4 times).

Stems

A A 45-year-old lady with a previous history of cancer in one breast.
B A 75-year-old lady who is normally healthy and fit.
C A post-menopausal woman, who is nulliparous and her BMI is 40.
D A 45-year-old woman whose 40-year-old sister has recently been diagnosed with breast cancer.
E A 49-year-old woman who has been on hormone replacement therapy for 10 years.

Question 3. Diagnosis of breast disease - breast imaging

Options

1 No imaging required.
2 No further imaging required.
3 Ultrasound scan (USS).
4 Mammography.
5 Magnetic resonant imaging (MRI).

Stems

A A 30-year-old woman presents with a discrete breast lump.
B A 25-year-old girl presents with cyclical pain, but no clinical abnormalities on examination.
C A 49-year-old woman has got thickening in the left upper quadrant but no discrete lump.

D A 39-year-old woman presents with pain in both breasts, no palpable abnormality on examination and mammography is normal.

E A 55-year-old woman with a clinically malignant lump; there is a suspicion on mammography and ultrasound scanning of multifocality.

F A 33-year-old woman with a suspicious lump on clinical examination and a normal/benign USS.

G A 60-year-old woman with a thickened area at the site of a previous wide local excision, and mammogram and USS are inconclusive.

Question 4. Diagnosis of breast disease - cytology report of fine needle aspirate

Options

1 C1.
2 C2.
3 C3.
4 C4.
5 C5.

Stems

A Definitely benign.
B Definitely malignant.
C Probably benign.
D Suspicious of malignancy.
E Inadequate.

Question 5. Diagnosis of breast disease - core biopsy classification

Options

1 B1.
2 B2.
3 B3.
4 B4.
5 B5.

Stems

A Definitely benign.
B Definitely malignant.
C Probably benign.
D Suspicious of malignancy.
E Normal breast tissue or no lesion identified.

Question 6. Diagnosis of breast disease - breast biopsy

Options

1 No biopsy required.
2 Fine needle aspirate cytology (FNAC)/Core biopsy.
3 Excision biopsy.
4 Excision biopsy after image guidance.
5 Vacuum assisted biopsy.

Stems

A A 30-year-old with a discrete lump, solid on USS and clinically thought to be fibroadenoma
B A 49-year-old lady with a thickened area in the right upper quadrant, but normal mammogram and USS.
C A 28-year-old woman presents with pain in both breasts, but clinical examination and USS are both normal.

D   A 45-year-old lady with a palpable lump, which is suspicious on mammogram and USS, but benign on core biopsy.

E   A 53-year-old lady with suspicious microcalcification on a screening mammogram. Examination and USS are normal and stereotactic core biopsy reveals benign calcification only.

Question 7. Diagnosis of breast disease - breast biopsy

Options

1   Reassure and discharge.
2   Clinical follow-up.
3   Excision biopsy.
4   Excision biopsy after image guidance.
5   Vacuum assisted biopsy.

Stems

A   A 55-year-old woman who had a lump excised from her breast. The diagnosis was a benign phyllodes tumour.

B   A 37-year-old female presents with cyclical pain. Nodular breasts but no discrete lump. USS and mammogram normal.

C   A 38-year-old woman underwent a core biopsy of a small, non-palpable mammographic abnormality. The biopsy results came back as typical of fibroadenoma, which correlated with the radiology.

D   A 37-year-old woman underwent biopsy of a small, non-palpable area of mammographic calcification. The biopsy results came back as showing atypical ductal hyperplasia.

E   A 40-year-old woman is found to have a 30mm firm smooth mass in the upper outer quadrant of the breast consistent with a simple cyst. The mass is aspirated, and 10mls of cloudy green fluid is removed.

F   A 38-year-old with a palpable and mammographic lump shown to be a complex cyst on ultrasound. Core biopsy was B1.

Question 8. Nipple discharge

Options

1 Fibrocystic breast disease.
2 Galactorrhoea.
3 Intraduct papilloma.
4 Breast cancer.
5 Mammary duct ectasia.

Stems

A A 39-year-old woman who has been taking methyldopa presents with milky discharge from both breasts.
B A 38-year-old female complains of bilateral green/brown nipple discharge associated with cyclical pain.
C A 42-year-old woman presents with unilateral persistent blood-stained nipple discharge.
D Measurements of serum prolactin is an appropriate investigation.
E A 55-year-old woman presents with pain in the nipple with intermittent blood-stained or creamy discharge.

Question 9. Nipple discharge

Options

1 Physiological.
2 Mammary duct fistula.
3 Cancer.
4 Intraductal papilloma.
5 Duct ectasia.

Stems

A A woman in her sixties presents with bloody discharge from the nipple. Attempts at expressing discharge by the examining clinician fail, but a mammogram reveals an area of microcalcification. USS shows no associated mass.

B   A multiparous woman in her forties presents with clear discharge from the breast. A mammogram and USS reveal no abnormality.

C   A woman in her fifties presents with a green nipple discharge. Breast imaging shows dilated and calcified ducts.

Question 10. The inflamed or swollen breast

Options

1   Peau d'orange.
2   Periductal mastitis.
3   Puerpueral mastitis.
4   Inflammatory carcinoma.
5   Galactocoele.

Stems

A   A woman presents 3 weeks postpartum with a painful swelling of her right breast. She is systemically unwell and on examination of the breast it is inflamed and swollen but there is no evidence of a mass.

B   A woman presents with painless enlargement of the right breast 6 weeks after she gave birth to a child with a cleft palate. On examination, the breast is enlarged, non-tender and there are no signs of inflammation.

C   An elderly woman presents with redness of the breast not associated with pain.

D   A patient known to have duct ectasia develops pain and redness around the nipple.

Question 11. Benign breast disorders

Options

1 Gynaecomastia.
2 Fibroadenoma.
3 Fat necrosis.
4 Papillomas.
5 Cysts.

Stems

A The most common tumour in women under the age of 30.
B Polyps of epithelial-lined breast ducts.
C Associated with some functioning testicular tumour.
D Changes in the menstrual cycle.
E Usually secondary to previous trauma and contain inflammatory cells.

Question 12. Breast disease - breast pain

Options

1 Referred pain.
2 Cyclical mastalgia.
3 Tietze's syndrome.
4 Duct ectasia.

Stems

A A 36-year-old lady presented with 3 weeks' history of left breast pain. On examination there is only a localised tenderness at the medial edge of the left breast.
B A 46-year-old woman presented with 6 weeks' history of burning pain centrally in the left breast and a history of nipple discharge. On examination there is central nipple retraction and subareolar tenderness.

C   A 32-year-old woman presented with bilateral breast pain for 3 months worse during the second half of her menstrual cycle. On examination there is bilateral tenderness in both upper outer quadrants.

D   A 64-year-old woman has longstanding persistent pain in the upper outer quadrant of the right breast. The pain radiates down her arm and she has pain in her neck.

Question 13. Breast diseases

Options

1   Paget's disease.
2   Fibroadenoma.
3   Breast cyst.
4   Breast carcinoma.
5   Mammary duct ectasia.
6   Mammary duct fistula.
7   Traumatic fat necrosis.

Stems

A   A 47-year-old woman has been aware of a painful right nipple for 2 months. For the last 2 weeks, she has been aware of a discharge from that nipple. Since then, the pain has been less severe. When you examine her you notice a purulent discharge can be expressed from a single opening at the outer margin of the areola.

B   A 69-year-old woman who complains of an itch affecting the right nipple over the last 4 months. She attends because she has noticed some 'crusting' over the nipple and a discharge which stains her bra.

C   A 35-year-old woman who presents having been a passenger in a car which was involved in a road accident. She was wearing a seat belt and sustained bruising of the breast due to the restraining effect of the seat belt. A lump appeared in the breast at the site of bruising but both bruising and lump subsequently disappeared.

Question 14. TNM classification of breast cancer

Options

1   T2N1M0.
2   T2N2M0.
3   T2N1M1.
4   T4N3M0.
5   T4N1M0.

Stems

A   A 36-year-old women who is breast feeding has noticed that her right breast is red, swollen and hard. She has not responded to a course of antibiotics given by her GP. At the breast clinic, triple assessment reveals an 80mm carcinoma centrally, with some mobile nodes in the ipsilateral axilla.

B   A 64-year-old women presents to the breast clinic having ignored a lump of 30mm in her left upper outer quadrant with skin fixation. There are palpable nodes in the left axilla and supraclavicular fossa.

C   A 53-year-old woman presents to the breast clinic with a 25mm tumour in the right upper inner quadrant. Hard fixed matted nodes are found in the right axilla.

Question 15. TNM classification of breast cancer

Each of the following patients has breast cancer with a normal chest x-ray and blood chemistries; none has bone pain.

Options

1   T1N1M0.
2   T2N0M1.
3   T4N2M0.
4   T2N0M0.
5   T4N1M0.

Stems

A Mobile 15mm primary tumour with no skin involvement, but associated with a 20mm hard mobile axillary lymph node on the same side.

B Mobile 40mm primary tumour with no skin involvement. Both axillary and supraclavicular lymph nodes are normal.

C 55mm primary tumour associated with peau d'orange appearance of the overlying skin and a 10mm hard mobile axillary lymph node on the same side.

D Mobile 30mm primary tumour with no skin involvement and normal axillary lymph nodes, but associated with a 10mm hard supraclavicular lymph node.

E 20mm primary tumour associated with skin ulceration and hard matted, but mobile axillary lymph nodes on the same side.

Question 16. Staging of breast cancer

Options

1 UICC I.
2 UICC II.
3 UICC III.
4 UICC IV.

Stems

A 15mm tumour. No palpable lymph nodes.
B 32mm tumour. Mobile axillary lymph node.
C Fungating tumour. No metastases.
D 41mm tumour. Boney metastases.

Question 17. Breast carcinoma

Options

1   Late menopause.
2   Is the most accurate predictor of outcome.
3   Lobular carcinoma *in situ*.
4   Multifocal carcinoma *in situ*.
5   Late menarche.
6   Ductal carcinoma *in situ*.

Stems

A   Nodal status.
B   There is no mammograpgic abnormalities.
C   Paget's disease of the nipple is associated with ...
D   Usually treated with mastectomy.
E   Considered as a risk factor for developing breast cancer.

Question 18. Breast cancer

Options

1   Male breast cancer.
2   Female breast cancer.
3   Both male and female breast cancer.
4   Neither male nor female breast cancer.

Stems

A   Tamoxifen is a mainstay of hormonal therapy.
B   Present primarily as a subareolar mass.
C   5-year survival independent of stage.
D   Tumour size a prognostic factor.

Question 19. Pathological types of breast cancer and associated features

Options

1   Infiltrating ductal carcinoma.
2   Ductal carcinoma *in situ.*
3   Lobular carcinoma *in situ.*
4   Phyllodes tumour.
5   Inflammatory carcinoma.

Stems

A   Often large but quite mobile.
B   Highest likelihood of multicentric ipsilateral disease.
C   Highest likelihood of bilateral disease.
D   Dermal lymphatic invasion.
E   Most common carcinoma presenting a breast mass.

Question 20. Surgical treatment of breast cancer

Options

1   Total mastectomy +/- primary reconstruction.
2   Wide local excision with no axillary procedure.
3   Total mastectomy and axillary clearance.
4   Wide local excision and axillary staging.

Stems

A   A 46-year-old woman with diffuse microcalcification of the left breast, no masses palpable; stereotactic biopsy of two, 30mm clusters in the lower inner and lower outer quadrants shows low-grade ductal carcinoma *in situ* (DCIS).
B   A 68-year-old woman with a 55mm infiltrating ductal carcinoma in the lower inner left breast; mass large enough to disrupt the contour of her small breast, but no skin changes; solitary 20mm lymph node palpable in the left axilla.

C   A 51-year-old woman with a 20mm palpable mass in the upper outer quadrant of the left breast; core biopsy reveals comedo DCIS.

D   A 36-year-old woman with a 5mm focus of cribriform DCIS in the upper outer quadrant of the left breast; no palpable masses.

E   A 78-year-old woman with an 11mm tubular carcinoma in the lower outer quadrant of the right breast.

Question 21. Surgical treatment of breast disease

Options

1   Wide local excision with axillary dissection.
2   Re-excision with free margins and close follow-up.
3   Axillary dissection. No breast procedure.
4   No further surgery; close follow-up.
5   Total mastectomy without axillary dissection.

Stems

A   A 39-year-old woman underwent a surgical biopsy of a small, non-palpable mammographic abnormality. The biopsy results are typical of lobular carcinoma *in situ* and the resection edges are involved.

B   A smooth, rubbery 30mm lesion is removed from the breast of a 35-year-old woman with a pre-operative diagnosis of fibroadenoma. Histologically, this lesion is found to be a phyllodes tumour which reaches the margins of excision.

C   A 72-year-old woman presents with multifocal invasive lobular carcinoma.

D   A 52-year-old woman presents with a mobile lymph node in the left axilla. Core biopsy confirms invasive carcinoma consistent with breast primary. Examination and imaging of the breast reveals no primary and staging is normal.

Question 22. Treatment of breast cancer

Options

1 Primary chemotherapy.
2 Wide local excision and axillary staging.
3 Total mastectomy +/- reconstruction.
4 Total mastectomy and axillary staging.
5 Primary hormonal treatment.

Stems

A An 88-year-old woman presents with a firm 25mm lump in the right lower breast. Core biopsy shows B5 with oestrogen receptor positive.

B A 37-year-old woman presents with a 45mm lump in the left axillary tail. Nodes palpable in the axilla. Core biopsy confirms invasive ductal carcinoma.

C A 51-year-old female with widespread microcalcification noted throughout the breast on screening mammography. Multiple core biopsies show DCIS but no invasive disease.

D A 66-year-old female with an ulcerated right nipple. No lump palpable. Nipple biopsy shows Paget's disease.

E A 53-year-old woman with a 20mm diameter lump in the right axillary tail. Core biopsy confirms carcinoma.

Question 23. Axillary surgery in breast cancer

Options

1 No axillary surgery.
2 Axillary staging.
3 Axillary clearance.

Stems

A   A 57-year-old woman with a cluster of microcalcification noted on
     screening mammography. Core biopsies show DCIS but no
     invasive disease.

B   A 48-year-old woman presents with a 40mm lump in the left
     breast. Nodes are palpable in the axilla. Core biopsy confirms
     invasive ductal carcinoma.

C   A 62-year-old woman with a 20mm diameter lump in the right
     breast. Core biopsy confirms invasive ductal carcinoma.

D   A 53-year-old woman presents with a 30mm palpable mass in the
     upper half of the right breast. Core biopsy reveals comedo DCIS
     with microinvasion.

Question 24. Anatomy of the axilla

Options

1   Anterior wall.
2   Posterior wall.
3   Lateral wall.
4   Medial wall.

Stems

A   Pectoralis major.
B   Humerus.
C   Latissimus dorsi.
D   Subscapularis.
E   Serratus anterior.

Question 25. Axillary dissection

Options

1   Serratus anterior muscle.
2   Long thoracic nerve.
3   Intercostobrachial nerve.
4   Subscapularis muscle.
5   Thoracodorsal nerve.
6   Pectoralis minor.

Stems

A   A 45-year-old woman on examination post-left mastectomy and axillary clearance, was found to have a winged scapula on the left side.
B   The medial wall of the axilla is formed by ...
C   A 50-year-old woman underwent a right mastectomy and axillary clearance. On the following outpatient appointment she complained about an anaesthetic patch on the upper medial aspect of her right arm.
D   In axillary lymph node dissection, level II nodes are those lying behind ...
E   The posterior wall of the axilla is formed by latissimus dorsi and ...

Question 26. Adjuvant systematic treatments in breast cancer

Options

1   None.
2   Hormonal only.
3   Chemotherapy only.
4   Both hormonal and chemotherapy.

Stems

A   A 62-year-old woman with a 30mm node negative, grade 3 tumour; oestrogen receptor (ER)-negative and progesterone receptor (PR)-negative.

B   A 69-year-old woman with an 18mm node negative, grade 1 and ER-positive.

C   A 59-year-old woman with a 15mm node negative, grade 2 and ER-negative breast carcinoma.

D   A 58-year-old woman with a 34mm node positive, grade 2 and ER-positive.

E   A 55-year-old woman with a 25mm node negative, grade 3 and ER-positive.

F   A 57-year-old woman with a 6mm node negative, grade 1 and ER-positive.

Question 27. Adjuvant hormonal treatments in breast cancer

Options

1   None.
2   Tamoxifen.
3   Aromatase inhibitor (Anastrozole).
4   Luteinising hormone releasing hormone analogue (Goserelin).

Stems

A   A 66-year-old woman with a 23mm breast tumour, grade 3, node negative and ER-positive.

B   A 60-year-old woman with a 6mm tubular carcinoma, grade 1, node negative and ER-negative.

C   A 65-year-old woman who had surgery for ER-positive breast cancer but has a history of previous pulmonary embolus.

D   A 38-year-old woman with a 15mm node negative, grade 2 and ER-positive breast tumour.

Question 28. Primary medical treatments in breast cancer

Options

1   Tamoxifen.
2   Aromatase inhibitor.
3   Chemotherapy.
4   Radiotherapy.

Stems

A   A 52-year-old woman with inflammatory breast carcinoma.
B   A 76-year-old woman presents with a locally advanced ER-positive tumour.
C   An 80-year-old woman with operable, ER-positive breast cancer who declines surgery because of a previous stroke.
D   A 53-year-old woman with a large operable tumour and who wants to avoid mastectomy.

Question 29. Radiotherapy treatment in breast cancer

Options

1   No radiotherapy.
2   Radiotherapy to breast.
3   Radiotherapy to chest wall.
4   Radiotherapy to axilla.
5   Radiotherapy to supraclavicular fossa.

Stems

A   A 52-year-old woman with a 29mm node negative invasive duct carcinoma who had undergone wide local excision (WLE) and axillary staging.
B   A 61-year-old woman with a small cluster of low-grade ductal carcinoma *in situ* (DCIS) treated by WLE with good clear margins.

C   A 64-year-old woman with a cluster of high-grade DCIS treated by WLE with good clear margins.

D   A 70-year-old woman with a 38mm tumour, treated by mastectomy and axillary sampling which revealed 2 positive lymph nodes out of the 4 sampled.

E   A 65-year-old woman with a 55mm grade 2 lobular carcinoma treated by mastectomy and axillary clearance; more than 3 axillary lymph nodes were positive.

Question 30. Correlation of response to hormonal therapy with ER/PR status

Options

1   80%.
2   45%.
3   35%.
4   10%.

Stems

A   ER-positive/PR-negative.
B   ER-positive/PR-positive.
C   ER-negative/PR-positive.
D   ER-negative/PR-negative.

Question 31. Nottingham prognostic index

Options

1 <3.
2 <3.4.
3 3.4-5.4.
4 >5.4.

Stems

A Excellent prognosis.
B Poor prognosis.
C Intermediate prognosis.
D Good prognosis.

Answer 1   A4, B1, C1, D3, E1

Benign breast conditions due to aberrations in normal development and involution (ANDI), such as sclerosing adenosis, duct ectasia, fibroadenoma and cysts, are not associated with any increased risk of developing malignant changes. Epithelial hyperplasia without atypia is associated with slight increased risk, whilst atypical ductal hyperplasia and atypical lobular hyperplasia are associated with moderate increased risk. Lobular carcinoma *in situ* is considered a marker of underlying risk of developing breast cancer.

Answer 2   A4, B4, C2, D3, E2

Age is the greatest risk factor for breast cancer, with the relative risk increasing with increasing age. Only 10% of breast cancers are due to genetic predisposition, with half attributed to mutations in the BRCA1 or BRCA2 gene. A previous history of cancer in the other breast or a strong family history are associated with high relative risk (>4) eg. two first degree relatives who developed breast cancer at an early age. History of high-dose radiation to the chest or one first degree relative diagnosed with breast cancer under 40 years is associated with a moderate relative risk (2.1-4.0). Factors associated with a low relative risk (1.1-2.0) include: age at first full-term pregnancy >30 years, age at menarche <12 years, age at menopause >50 years, obesity, nulliparity in post-menopausal women and use of hormonal contraceptives when young. Hormone replacement therapy taken for longer than 5 years is associated with a low relative risk but combined hormone replacement therapy may carry more relative risk than preparations containing oestrogen only.

Answer 3   A3, B1, C4, D2, E5, F4, G5

Triple assessment with a combination of clinical examination, breast imaging and needle biopsy forms the basis of diagnosis of breast disease. Mammography is the first imaging of choice in patients over 35 years, with ultrasonography used also if there is a clinical and/or mammographic abnormality. For women under 35 years, ultrasonography is the first imaging but if there is a clinical or ultrasonographic suspicion these patients should also proceed to mammography. Mammography should always be undertaken in women with breast cancer to check for multifocality, calcification associated with DCIS and to check the contralateral breast. Mammography has a positive predictive value for cancers of 95% and this figure rises to 98% when combined with ultrasonography. Full field digital mammography and high frequency ultrasound have increased the diagnostic accuracy of breast imaging in both benign and malignant breast disease. MRI may be particularly helpful in ascertaining multifocality of a cancer or in detecting recurrent cancer in the breast following previous treatment.

Answer 4   A2, B5, C3, D4, E1

Fine needle aspiration cytology (FNAC) is cheap and the result may be available quickly whilst the patient is in the breast clinic. However, it requires an experienced cytopathologist and despite high sensitivity for breast cancer there may be inadequate or equivocal results. Such patients require further biopsy procedures, usually core biopsy. FNAC which is C1 'inadequate', i.e. showing no epithelial cells, may be diagnostic in certain circumstances such as fat necrosis or lipoma where there are macrophages and fat cells respectively.

Answer 5   A2, B5, C3, D4, E1

Core biopsy using 14 or 16 gauge needles is now becoming the
needle biopsy procedure of choice, where it is often used with image
guidance. It provides more information about the diagnosis, especially
breast cancer, where the type, predicted grade and ER status may be
ascertained prior to treatment. This is particularly important in patients
undergoing primary medical treatment. More recently, vacuum assisted
percutaneous biopsy, (eg. Mammotome) has been introduced. It uses
a larger needle, 8 or 11 gauge, under suction to obtain larger amounts
of tissue for the pathologist. It is therefore superior to core biopsy in
discriminating between the diagnosis of ADH and DCIS, or between
DCIS and invasive cancer. It is also being used for treatment of benign
conditions such as fibroadenoma or gynaecomastia.

Answer 6   A2, B2, C1, D3 & 5, E4 & 5

Answer 7   A2, B1, C1, D4 & 5, E1, F3

Needle biopsy should be undertaken as part of the triple assessment
when there is a clinical and/or radiological abnormality. Where there is
correlation between the clinico-radiological findings and the needle
biopsy, decisions regarding the definitive management of patients may
be made. Many patients may be discharged, eg. simple cyst or
fibroadenoma, or put into follow-up protocols, eg. ADH or benign
phyllodes, where there is a risk of local recurrence. If however, there is
no correlation then a further test should be undertaken. This would
normally be the next test in sequence, FNAC, core biopsy, open biopsy.
With the advent of vacuum assisted biopsy however, excision biopsy
may be avoided. Where the core biopsy is B3 or B4, eg. ADH, either a
vacuum assisted biopsy or excision biopsy with or without image
guidance should be undertaken. Complex cysts diagnosed on
ultrasound should be excised.

Answer 8   A2, B1, C3 & 4, D2, E3 & 4

Answer 9   A3, B1, C5

Galactorrhoea is milk secretion unrelated to breast feeding, usually bilateral and can occur spontaneously. Causes of galactorrhoea include:

1. Physiological (post-lactation, stress).
2. Drugs (those associated with hyperprolactinaemia; [eg. phenothiazines, haloperidol, methyldopa] and others [eg. oestrogens, opiates]).
3. Pathological (eg. hypothalamic and pituitary stalk lesion, pituitary tumours, ectopic prolactin secretion, hypothyroidism, chronic renal failure).

Blood-stained discharges are most likely due to papilloma, where the discharge is single duct and persistent, or duct ectasia, where the bleeding is intermittent. Bleeding from the nipple as a sole symptom is rarely due to breast cancer. Fibrocystic disease usually affects women between 35-45 years of age. This term encompasses the triad of pain, nodularity and cyst formation in the female breast. The discharge associated with this condition is usually green/brown in colour. Mammary duct ectasia also causes a creamy or green discharge. Green discharge can also happen around menopause. Ultrasound is particularly helpful in the assessment of duct discharge but ductography and cytology of duct lavage may also be used.

Answer 10   A3, B5, C4, D2

Patients who develop mastitis and breast abscess following breast feeding are often systemically unwell with few localising signs in the breast. Periductal mastitis secondary to duct ectasia may be treated with antibiotics and percutaneous aspiration, thus minimising the risk of mamillary fistula. Galactocoele can be treated by aspiration and suppressing lactation. Inflammatory carcinoma is often mistaken for mastitis but is usually painless.

Answer 11   A2, B4, C1, D5, E3

Fibroadenoma is the most common tumour in women under the age of 30. They present with a firm, mobile painless lump. Many fibroadenomas get smaller or disappear. Gynaecomastia is a benign hypertrophy of the breast disc and may have a hormonal basis. Gynaecomastia of puberty usually settles spontaneously. In older males, bilateral gynaecomastia may result from excess circulating oestrogen due to liver disease, certain testicular tumours or drugs such as cimetidine, diazepam or spironolactone. Trauma to the breast, sometimes trivial or even unnoticed, may cause necrosis of adipose issue. Initially, there is an acute inflammatory response but if necrotic fat remains, the inflammatory picture becomes more chronic. A papilloma should be excised by microdochectomy.

Answer 12   A3, B4, C2, D1

Breast pain (mastalgia) is the most common breast-related complaint among women. There are two main types of breast pain: cyclical and non-cyclical. Cyclical breast pain accounts for nearly 75% of all breast complaints. Of all women who experience breast pain, two thirds experience cyclical breast pain. Though cyclical breast pain is usually related to the menstrual cycle, stress may also affect hormone levels and influence breast pain. Non-cyclical breast pain is far less common and is not related to a woman's menstrual cycle. Non-cyclical breast pain is most common in women between 40 and 50 years of age. The pain is often described as burning and is typically associated with underlying benign breast change such as duct ectasia. Other factors that may contribute to breast pain in some women include: oral contraceptive pills, hormone replacement therapy, weight gain, underwired or ill-fitting brassiere. Non-cyclical pain may arise from the chest wall eg. costochondritis or Tietze's syndrome. Cervical spondylosis may cause referred pain in the breast but is often associated with pain down the arm and paraesthesia in the fingers. All women must be properly assessed but most women with moderate breast pain are not treated with medications or surgical procedures. Advice and reassurance are usually enough. Drug treatment is indicated only in certain cases where breast pain is severe and interferes with a woman's daily activities; gamolenic acid (GLA), found in evening primrose oil or starflower oil is the first-line medication for cyclical mastalgia. Danazol or bromocriptine may be used if GLA is not effective after 3 months' treatment.

Answer 13   A5, B1, C7

Mammary duct fistula: this history is in keeping with an episode of sepsis in the nipple which has resolved when the infected material spontaneously discharged through the skin at the areolar margin. The identification of a discharging sinus at the outer margin of the nipple areolar confirms the diagnosis of a mammary duct fistula. There is usually a consequence of periductal mastitis secondary to duct ectasia. Paget's disease: this history bears the hallmark of Paget's disease - a nipple itch, eczematous changes in the nipple, areola and surrounding skin, together with bleeding or discharges from the nipple. These changes are associated with an underlying invasive or *in situ* breast cancer. Fat necrosis occurs after trauma to the breast. Whilst the condition usually resolves spontaneously, the lump may be hard and craggy, thus mimicking the features of a breast cancer.

Answer 14   A5, B3, C2

Answer 15   A1, B4, C5, D2, E3

Clinical staging is assessed using the tumour node metastases (TNM) classification. There is also a separate TNM classification using pathological measurements. T is for tumour size: *Tis* is for carcinoma *in situ*, T1 is for tumour less than 20mm; T2 between 20 and 50mm; T3 larger than 50mm and T4 is any tumour size with fixation to the chest wall or skin. N is for lymph nodes: N0 axillary lymph nodes not involved, N1 ipsilateral mobile axillary nodal metastases, N2 ipsilateral matted or fixed axillary nodal metastases, N3 ipsilateral internal mammary nodal metastases. M is for metastases: M0 no metastases and M1 is for distant metastases. Supraclavicular nodal metastases (formerly considered to be N3 are now thought to represent distant metastases M1).

Answer 16   A1, B2, C3, D4

The UICC (International Union Against Cancer) staging incorporates the TNM system of staging. T <2cm, N0, M0 = stage I, T = 2-5cm, N 0-I, M0 = stage II, and T3, T4 or N2-3 = stage 3, distant metastasis = stage IV.

Answer 17   A2, B3, C6, D4, E1

Factors associated with an increased risk of developing breast cancer include: first degree relatives (5% of breast cancer is inherited and linked to two genes: BRCA1 and BRCA2), early menarche, late menopause, oral contraceptive pill/hormonal replacement therapy and obesity. Axillary nodal status and the number of metastatic lymph nodes are the most important factors with regard to survival. Lobular carcinoma *in situ* is a pre-invasive breast cancer usually diagnosed incidentally as it is not palpable and has no specific mammographic features. It usually affects pre-menopausal women and tends to be multifocal and bilateral. Paget's disease of the breast is generally considered to be primary ductal carcinoma that secondarily invades the epithelium of the nipple and areola. Therefore, it typically presents with eczematous rash involving the nipple and areola. Paget's disease is usually associated with an intraductal carcinoma or an infiltrating carcinoma with or without a palpable mass.

Answer 18   A3, B1, C4, D3

One percent of all breast cancers occur in men. Breast cancer in men affects predominantly older patients with a peak incidence of 60 years of age. Most male breast cancers (75%-95%) present as a painless subareolar mass while this is a much less common location for breast cancer in females. Very few present with pain or nipple discharge. Increasing tumour size and involvement of axillary lymph nodes have a negative impact on patient survival, and the stage of the tumour at presentation correlates with the 5-year survival in both men and women. Approximately 65% to 85% of male breast cancers are oestrogen receptor positive and 67% are progesterone receptor positive. Hormonal manipulation is appropriate in the management of male breast cancer, just as in female breast cancer.

Answer 19   A4, B2, C3, D5, E1.

Ductal carcinoma *in situ* (DCIS) is frequently found as an area of clustered microcalcifications on the mammogram and uncommonly presents as a palpable mass. Comedo DCIS is associated with a high incidence of multicentricity while non-comedo DCIS tends to be more localised. Lobular carcinoma *in situ* usually presents as an incidental histological finding at biopsy of another lesion in pre-menopausal women. Its significance is that it is a marker of malignancy with an approximately 25-30% chance of developing an invasive carcinoma within 15 years of diagnosis, with both breasts being at essentially equal risk. Inflammatory carcinoma, a variant of infiltrating ductal carcinoma, is characterised by the clinical appearance of inflammation (peau d'orange and erythema) secondary to dermal lymphatic invasion. Cystosarcoma phyllodes resembles a giant fibroadenoma clinically and histologically, and it occurs in both benign and malignant forms. If benign, adequate treatment consists of total excision with adequate (>1cm) margins. Long-term follow-up is mandatory, as recurrences are not uncommon and can be of the malignant variety. If malignant usually requires mastectomy to achieve local control.

Answer 20   A1, B3, C2, D2, E4

The primary operative goals for the management of breast cancer remain local control of the primary tumour and regional staging of the disease. Overall, breast conserving therapy is possible in up to 70% of patients. Large tumour to breast ratio, multifocal multiquadrant disease and personal preference may prevent a breast preserving operation. Patient A requires total mastectomy because of multiquadrant disease. Patient B requires total mastectomy because of her high tumour-to-breast volume ratio. Patient C can be managed with wide local excision to free margins and postoperative radiotherapy to decrease the risk of local recurrence. Management of patients with minimal focus of DCIS, as in patient D, is controversial at this time. This low-grade tumour may require excision alone, without radiotherapy, if surgical margins are clear. Most authors would advise against radiotherapy for this small lesion. Adjuvant tamoxifen may be given for chemoprevention of the contralateral breast. In patient E wide local excision with axillary staging and breast irradiation is an appropriate treatment. Axillary staging is mandatory in invasive tumours but is not appropriate for *in situ* disease.

Answer 21   A4, B2, C5, D3

Lobular carcinoma *in situ* is associated with a 9-fold increase in the likelihood of developing invasive breast cancer. There is no need to obtain free margins because it does not decrease the risk. Even if the margins are involved, the cancer that may subsequently develop is no more likely to occur at the site of the biopsy than at any other site in either breast. Patients should be followed-up in accordance with breast cancer follow-up protocols. Phyllodes tumours have a tendency to recur locally and should also be followed-up. Patients presenting with axillary lymphadenopathy should be staged to exclude metastases. If imaging of the breast, including MRI, shows no primary, the breast may be treated by radiotherapy or mastectomy.

Answer 22   A5, B1 & B4, C3, D4, E2

Excision of the tumour remains the mainstay of treatment regardless of age. In elderly patients who are unfit or unwilling to undergo surgery, hormonal manipulation may be given if the tumour is ER and/or PgR positive. Surgical treatment is either by wide local excision (breast-conserving surgery) plus radiotherapy, or mastectomy (with or without reconstruction). Axillary staging is at present necessary for all cases of invasive carcinoma, but not in DCIS. For women presenting with an operable tumour too large for breast conservation, pre-operative (neoadjuvant) chemotherapy may be given to 'downsize' the lesion, thus allowing subsequent breast conservation and the avoidance of mastectomy.

Answer 23   A1, B3, C2, D1

Axillary staging is not necessary in patients with DCIS or microinvasion. If there are palpable nodes in the axilla they should be treated with clearance. For other patients with invasive disease and no evidence of axillary lymphadenopathy the axilla should be staged. This may be done by clearance or four node sampling. If the four node sampling proves positive, the axilla should be treated by radiotherapy or proceeding to full clearance. The risk for axillary metastases increases with the size and primary features of the primary tumour, including histological grade and vascular invasion, ranging from 0-20% for T1 lesions and up to 50% for T2 lesions. Certain tumour types, including tubular carcinomas, rarely metastasize to axillary lymph nodes. The technique of sentinel node sampling is likely to replace axillary clearance as a staging tool, thereby avoiding the morbidity of clearance, such as lymphoedema and shoulder stiffness.

Answer 24   A1, B3, C2, D2, E4

The axilla is a fat-filled space. Its shape is that of a truncated pyramid with apex, base and four sides. The medial wall is formed by the ribs and serratus anterior, the lateral by the humerus, the anterior by pectoralis major and minor, and the posterior by subscapularis and latissimus dorsi.

Answer 25   A2, B1, C3, D6, E4

The thoracodorsal nerve supplies latissimus dorsi and the long thoracic nerve supplies serratus anterior. Division of the long thoracic nerve produces a winged scapula. Both nerves should be carefully dissected and preserved in axillary dissection. Level I nodes lie lateral to pectoralis minor, level II behind and level III medial to the muscle. Division of the intercostobrachial nerve leads to anaesthetic skin in the axilla and upper medial part of the arm.

Answer 26   A3, B2, C3, D4, E4, F1 & F2

While surgery and radiation offer local control of the primary tumour, systemic therapies aim to prevent or delay the appearance of distant metastases. This systemic treatment is called 'adjuvant' therapy and marks the most significant change in breast cancer management of the past 20 years. Hormonal adjuvant treatment is only effective in ER and/or PgR positive tumours. Where the prognosis of the patient is excellent there is controversy as to whether hormonal treatment should be given, bearing in mind the potential side effects. Cytotoxic chemotherapy is indicated in most ER/PgR negative tumours, the presence of grade 3 or positive axillary lymph nodes. Chemotherapy is more effective in pre-menopausal patients. The proportional reduction in annual mortality is reduced by 30% with combined chemotherapy and hormonal treatment in both pre- and post-menopausal women.

Answer 27   A2, B1, C3, D4

Currently, tamoxifen is the standard adjuvant hormonal treatment with anastrozole being prescribed where tamoxifen is contraindicated as in patient C. The side effects of tamoxifen on coagulation and the circulation make it inappropriate for patients with a previous history of thromboembolism, myocardial infarct or stroke. Goserelin, a luteinising hormone releasing hormone analogue, may be used in pre-menopausal women.

Answer 28   A3, B1 & 4, C2, D3

Primary medical treatment may be offered in locally advanced disease where downstaging the disease reduces the risk of local recurrence following subsequent mastectomy. Hormonal treatment is recommended in patients over 70 years with ER/PgR positive tumours, with women under 70 years or with ER/PgR negative tumours being offered chemotherapy. Primary medical treatment with chemotherapy may be used as a neoadjuvant treatment to avoid mastectomy in patients with a large operable tumour.

Answer 29   A2, B1, C2, D4, E3 & 5

Radiotherapy should be given to the breast in all patients undergoing wide local excision for invasive disease and those with intermediate or high-grade DCIS. Radiotherapy to the breast may be omitted in patients with low-grade DCIS who have had a wide local excision with adequate margins of clearance. Patients with positive sampling of the axilla need axillary treatment. This may be by giving radiotherapy or proceeding to a formal axillary clearance. The morbidity of surgery and radiotherapy to the axilla is similar but there may be a small survival advantage to surgical clearance. The indications for radiotherapy after mastectomy and axillary clearance are involvement of muscle or >3 positive axillary lymph nodes. The presence of a high-grade tumour or vascular invasion are more controversial indications. Radiotherapy to the supraclavicular fossa is indicated if >3 positive axillary lymph nodes. Radiotherapy to the axilla should be avoided after axillary clearance because of the high risk of lymphoedema.

Answer 30   A3, B1, C2, D4

Normal breast cells have receptors for oestrogen, progesterone, androgen and corticosteroids. Many breast cancers retain these receptors. In general, if receptors are present, the tumour has to some degree retained the regulatory mechanisms operating in normal breast epithelium. Their absence therefore, implies less controlled growth and a poorer overall prognosis. The increased response rate seen in some breast cancer subtypes with positive receptors provides the basis for endocrine manipulation, both additive and ablative. The most responsive receptor status is ER-positive/PR-positive followed by ER-negative/PR-positive, ER-positive/PR-negative, and ER-negative/PR-negative.

Answer 31   A1, B4, C3, D2

Adjuvant treatment is now based on prognostic factors within the tumour and regional nodes rather than on TNM or UICC staging. The important factors determining outcome are tumour size, status of the axillary lymph nodes, histological type of tumour, histological grade, lymphovascular invasion and hormone receptor status. The Nottingham prognostic index (NPI) uses tumour size, grade and lymph node status to predict outcome. The index is (the tumour size in cm x 0.2) + (grade) + (lymph node status), where no nodes involved = 0, 1-3 = 2 and >3 positive lymph nodes = 3. The studies looked at 'overall survival' (OS) at 15 years post-diagnosis (OS: 80%, 42% and 13% for NPI <3.4, 3.4-5.4, and >5.4 respectively). In order to calculate the index, axillary lymph node status must be known.

Chapter 8

Endocrine disease

Michele E Lucarotti, MD FRCS
Consultant Surgeon, Gloucestershire Royal Hospital, Gloucester, UK

For all questions each option may be used once, more than once or not at all.

Question 1. Thyroid surgery

Choose the most suitable management strategy for the following patients.

Options

1   Papillary carcinoma less than 10mm in diameter.
2   Hurthle cell tumour.
3   Minimally invasive follicular carcinoma.
4   Invasive follicular carcinoma.
5   Papillary carcinoma greater than 10mm in diameter.

Stems

A   Total thyroidectomy and radioactive I131 and thyroxine.
B   Total thyroidectomy and thyroxine alone.
C   Thyroxine alone.
D   Total thyroidectomy alone.
E   Total lobectomy including isthmusectomy.

Question 2. Thyroid surgery anatomy

Choose the correct function of the following nerves.

Options

1   Supplies all the muscles of the larynx except the crico thyroid and is sensory to the larynx below the vocal cords.
2   Is non-recurrent on the left side in 1% of cases.
3   Lies on the middle constrictor.
4   Supplies the crico thyroid and inferior constrictor.
5   80% lie medial to the superior thyroid artery.

Stems

A   The recurrent laryngeal nerve.
B   The superior laryngeal nerve.
C   The external laryngeal nerve.
D   The vagus nerve.
E   Non-recurrent laryngeal nerve.

Question 3. Multiple endocrine neoplasia syndromes

For each syndrome choose the commonly associated features.

Options

1   Most commonly associated with carcinoid tumours.
2   Marfanoid habitus.
3   Hyperplasia of the parathyroids.
4   Adreno-cortical tumours.
5   Phaeochromocytoma.

Stems

A   MEN I.
B   MEN IIa.
C   MEN IIb.
D   Sipple syndrome.
E   Wermer's syndrome.

Question 4. Carcinoid tumours of the appendix

For each of the clinical scenarios choose the most appropriate operation.

Options

1   Appendicectomy.
2   Right hemicolectomy if a fit patient.
3   Appendicectomy in a younger patient.
4   Right hemicolectomy in a younger patient.

Stems

A   Tumour greater than 2cm in size.
B   Involvement of mesoappendix.
C   Serosal involvement.
D   Involvement of intramucosal lymphatics.
E   Vascular invasion.

Question 5. Parathyroid glands

Choose the appropriate associated features of the following parathyroid sites.

Options

1   Third pharyngeal pouch.
2   Fourth pharyngeal pouch.
3   20% of cases.
4   Apex of thymus.
5   Tracheo-oesophageal groove.

Stems

A   The superior parathyroids.
B   The inferior parathyroids.
C   Intra-thyroidal parathyroids.
D   Ectopic superior parathyroid.
E   More than four parathyroids.

Question 6. Treatment of severe hypercalcaemia

Choose from the following options the appropriate treatment for hypercalcaemia in each of the following conditions.

Options

1   Hydration.
2   Biphosphanates.
3   Calcitonin.
4   Steroids.
5   Low calcium diet.

Stems

A   Malignancy.
B   Immobilisation.
C   Primary hyperparathyroidism.
D   Vitamin D intoxication.
E   Sarcoid.

Question 7. Management hypercalcaemia

For each of the following causes of hypercalcaemia, select the most appropriate description from the options listed.

Options

1   Commonest cause of hypercalcaemia in the population.
2   Commonest cause of hypercalcaemia in hospitals.
3   Severe symptomatic hypercalcaemia likely.
4   Related to parathyroid hormone-related peptide.
5   Causes hypercalcaemia mainly by increased calcium absorption due to increased level of 1, 25 - dihydroxy Vitamin D3.

Stems

A   Hyperparathyroidism.
B   Malignancy.
C   Vitamin D intoxication.
D   Sarcoidosis.
E   Immobilisation.

Question 8. Aetiology of thyroid disorders

For each of the following conditions select appropriate aetiologies.

Options

1   Hypothyroidism.
2   Graves disease.
3   Hyperthyroidism.
4   Painful thyroid.
5   Toxic multinodular goitre.

Stems

A   Radioactive iodine.
B   Sarcoidosis.
C   Hashimoto's thyroiditis.
D   DeQuervain's thyroiditis.
E   Metastatic thyroid carcinoma.

Question 9. Adrenal disorders

For the following disorders select associated features.

Options

1 Pituitary-dependent.
2 ACTH-dependent.
3 Exogenous steroids.
4 Increased skin pigmentation.
5 Visual field defects.

Stems

A Cushing's syndrome.
B Cushing's disease.
C Conn's syndrome.
D Nelson's syndrome.

Question 10. Adrenal tumours

For the following conditions choose common associations.

Options

1 Medullary thyroid carcinoma.
2 Neurofibromatosis.
3 Bilateral disease of the adrenal.
4 Increased urinary catecholamines.
5 Associated with increased serum ACTH.

Stems

A Phaeochromocytoma.
B Cushing's disease.
C Adreno-cortical carcinoma.
D Conn's syndrome.
E Adrenal lymphoma.

Answer 1   A2, B2, C5, D1, E1

Hurthle cell tumours are not radiosensitive. Differentiated carcinomas are treated by total thyroidectomy normally, except minimally invasive follicular carcinomas, which have an excellent prognosis with lobectomy only.

Answer 2   A1, B3 & 4, C3, 4 & 5, D1 & 4, E1

On the right side in 1% of cases the nerve is non-recurrent. On the left side the sixth branchial arch and hence sixth aortic artery persists as the ductus arteriosus preventing upward migration of the left recurrent laryngeal nerve. The superior laryngeal nerve divides into internal and external branches on the inferior constrictor.

Answer 3   A1, 3 & 4, B3 & 5, C2, 3 & 5, D2, 3 & 5, E1, 3 & 4

Wermer's syndrome is synomynous with MEN I and Sipple syndrome with MEN II. Although phaeochromocytomas are commonly associated with MEN II, adreno-cortical tumours are associated with MEN I.

Answer 4   A2 & 4, B4, C1, D1, E4

Appendicular carcinoids are rarely aggressive. Most tumours are at the tip. The major prognostic factor is the size of the original tumour. Metastatic disease is common with tumours greater than 2cm, but 98% of tumours are 1cm or less.

Answer 5   A2, B1 & 4, C1, D2, 3 & 5, E3

80% of superior glands are found within 1cm above the junction of the recurrent laryngeal nerve and inferior thyroid artery. In 80% of patients there are only four parathyroids. Ectopic superior glands may be found inferior to the inferior glands in the tracheo-oesophageal grove.

Answer 6 A1, 3 & 4, B1 & 3, C1, 3 & 5, D1, 3, 4 & 5, E1, 3, 4 & 5

Biphosphanates are poorly absorbed orally and should be given intravenously in severe cases. Calcitonin is an important agent in the early treatment of severe hypercalcaemia to obtain a rapid initial drop in serum calcium. Hypercalcaemia causes impaired glomerular filtration which is reduced further by volume depletion. Excretion of calcium is predominantly renal and this deterioration in glomerular filtration will adversely affect the body's ability to cope with an increased calcium load.

Steroids are only useful in reticulo-endothelial malignancy and sarcoid. Hyperparathyroidism will not respond to steroid therapy.

Dietary reduction of calcium is useful in primary hyperparathyroidism, sarcoid and Vitamin D intoxication, but not in malignancy.

Answer 7 A1, B2, 3 & 4, C4 & 5, E none

In most cases of malignancy causing hypercalcaemia, calcium absorption is suppressed due to a homeostatic reduction in 1, 25 - dihydroxy - Vitamin D production by the kidneys. The reverse situation is responsible for the hypercalcaemia in Vitamin D intoxication and sarcoid.

Answer 8 A1, B1, C1, 3 & 4, D3, E3

Hashimoto's thyroiditis can cause hyper- or hypothyroidism. Metastatic thyroid carcinoma is a rare cause of hyperthyroidism.

Answer 9 A1, 2 & 4, B1, 2 & 4, C1, D1, 2 & 4

Cushing's syndrome includes ACTH-dependent and independent causes of excess steroid production. ACTH-dependent Cushing's syndrome can then be sub-divided into ectopic and pituitary-dependent (Cushing's disease) types. Primary hyperaldosteronism may arise from an adrenal tumour (Conn's syndrome) or from bilateral adrenal hyperplasia. Nelson's syndrome occurs after bilateral adrenalectomy for Cushing's disease, when an unopposed pituitary tumour grows rapidly.

Answer 10   A1, 2, 3 & 4, B3 & 5, C none, D none, E3

Conn's syndrome is due to an adrenal tumour, although hyperaldosteronism can be due to bilateral adrenal hyperplasia. Adrenal adenomas tend to secrete a single steroid (cortisol or aldosterone). Carcinomas commonly secrete a wide variety of steroids often causing pronounced virilisation. Bilateral adrenal involvement is seen in 20% of phaeochromocytomas and 50% of adrenal lymphomas. Phaeochromocytomas and medullary thyroid carcinoma are part of the MEN II syndrome.

Chapter 9

Upper gastrointestinal surgery

Mark Vipond, MS FRCS

Consultant Surgeon, Gloucestershire Royal Hospital, Gloucester, UK

For all questions each option may be used once, more than once or not at all.

Oesophagogastric surgery

Question 1. Treatment of oesophageal neoplasia

In the following examples of oesophageal neoplasia select the most appropriate treatment.

Options

1   Radiotherapy.
2   Oesophageal resection.
3   Neoadjuvant chemotherapy and oesophageal resection.
4   Oesophageal stent.
5   Endoscopic mucosal resection.

Stems

A   A 55-year-old man with high-grade dysplasia in Barrett's oesophagus. Previous MI and insulin-dependent diabetes mellitus.
B   An 83-year-old lady with squamous cell carcinoma of middle third. Previous MI and COPD.

C   A 72-year-old man with adenocarcinoma of lower third. Staged by EUS as T3N1.

D   A 77-year-old man with adenocarcinoma of lower third. Total dysphagia and liver metastases.

E   A 64-year-old man with adenocarcinoma of lower third. Staged by EUS as T1N0.

Question 2. Dyspepsia

In the investigation and treatment of dyspepsia.

Options

1   Simple antacid or proton pump inhibitor (PPI).
2   Upper GI endoscopy.
3   13C urea breath test.
4   Barium meal.
5   Reassurance alone.

Stems

A   A 48-year-old man with a 3-month history of dyspepsia alone.

B   A 67-year-old man with a 6-week history of dyspepsia alone.

C   A 39-year-old man with a 3-month history of dyspepsia; also anaemia.

D   A 45-year-old women with a 6-week history of dyspepsia; normal upper GI endoscopy and treatment for *Helicobacter pylori* 6 months ago.

E   A 21-year-old women with a 6-month history of dyspepsia; no help with over the counter antacids.

Question 3. Staging

In the pathological staging of oesophagogastric cancer.

Options

1   TisN0M0.
2   T2N1M0.
3   T3N2M0.
4   T3N1M1a.
5   T4N3M1.

Stems

A   Carcinoma of distal third of oesophagus invading adventitia and involving para-oesophageal and coeliac nodes; no distant metastases.

B   Carcinoma of gastric antrum invading serosa, 8 nodes positive; no distant metastases.

C   Carcinoma of middle third of oesophagus, invading muscularis propria, 3 para-oesophageal nodes positive; no distant metastases.

D   Carcinoma of body of stomach without invasion of lamina propria and node negative.

E   Carcinoma of body of stomach invading pancreas, 17 nodes positive and peritoneal deposits.

Question 4. Management of gastro-oesophageal reflux disease

Options

1   Proton pump inhibitor (PPI).
2   Oesophageal dilatation.
3   Oesophageal resection.
4   Anti-reflux operation.
5   Photodynamic therapy.

Stems

A   A 59-year-old man, fit and well, with high-grade dysplasia in Barrett's on two separate endoscopic biopsies.

B   A 36-year-old man with non-neoplastic Barrett's and significant reflux with breakthrough symptoms on PPI.

C   An 83-year-old man with reflux and a recurrent benign oesophageal stricture.

D   A 45-year-old women with significant volume reflux, but poor oesophageal motility on stationary manometry.

E   A 68-year-old man with pH <4 for 6% of the time on a 24-hour pH study.

Question 5. Metabolic consequences of upper GI disease

Options

1   Fe-deficiency.
2   B_{12} deficiency.
3   Hypoalbuminaemia.
4   Hypokalaemia.
5   Vitamin D deficiency.

Stems

A   Ménétriere's disease.
B   Para-oesophageal hiatus hernia.
C   Gastric cancer.
D   Pyloric stenosis.
E   Patient 10 years post-gastrectomy.

Question 6. Acute upper GI haemorrhage

Options

1   Injection sclerotherapy.
2   Heater probe.
3   Rubber-band ligation.
4   Surgery.
5   Laser therapy.

Stems

A   A 65-year-old alcoholic man with oesophageal varices.
B   A 42-year-old man with a gastric ulcer; rebleed after injection.
C   A 64-year-old woman on aspirin; visible vessel in a duodenal ulcer.
D   A 54-year-old man with Dieulafoy's lesion.
E   A 32-year-old man with Mallory Weiss tear.

Question 7. Five-year survival for oesophagogastric cancer

Options

1   20%.
2   30%.
3   50%.
4   70%.
5   95%.

Stems

A   T1 N0 stomach.
B   T3 N1 oesophagus.
C   T2 N0 oesophagus.
D   T3 N2 stomach.
E   T3 N0 stomach.

Question 8. Dysphagia

Options

1 Achalasia.
2 Pharyngeal pouch.
3 Oesophageal neoplasm.
4 Benign peptic stricture.
5 Oesophageal dysmotility.

Stems

A A 74-year-old man with intermittent dysphagia, no weight loss and occasional regurgitation.

B A 65-year-old man with progressive dysphagia, weight loss of half a stone in two months and anorexia.

C An 81-year-old woman with dysphagia and regurgitation of unaltered food.

D A 65-year-old woman with dysphagia, weight loss of half a stone in two years and heartburn.

E A 30-year-old women with two years of dysphagia, some regurgitation and underweight.

Question 9. Surgery for gastric cancer

Options

1 Gastroenterostomy.
2 D1 partial gastrectomy.
3 D2 partial gastrectomy.
4 D2 total gastrectomy.
5 D2 total gastrectomy, splenectomy and distal pancreatectomy.

Stems

A A 65-year-old man with an obstructing tumour of the antrum; no metastases.

B A 73-year-old man with an obstructing tumour of the antrum; peritoneal deposits.

C   A 68-year-old man with a tumour of the body; no metastases.
D   A 66-year-old man with a tumour of the fundus, splenic artery nodes; no metastases.
E   A 68-year-old man with recurrent acute bleeding from a tumour of the antrum; peritoneal deposits.

Question 10. Oesophageal motility disorders

Match the oesophageal motility disorder to the stationary manometry findings.

Options

1   Scleroderma.
2   Achalasia.
3   Nutcracker oesophagus.
4   Diffuse oesophageal spasm.
5   Hypertensive lower oesophageal sphincter.

Stems

A   High amplitude and long contractions. Lower oesophageal sphincter (LOS) relaxes normally.
B   High amplitude contractions but normal peristalsis.
C   Decreased oesophageal contractions and low LOS pressure.
D   Aperistalsis and failure of LOS relaxation.
E   Normal peristalsis and contractions, but very high LOS pressure.

Question 11. Investigation

Select the appropriate investigation for the clinical scenario.

Options

1   CT scan.
2   Laparoscopy.
3   Endoluminal ultrasound (EUS).
4   Upper GI endoscopy.
5   Barium swallow.

Stems

A   An 84-year-old man with intermittent dysphagia and regurgitation of unaltered food.

B   A 64-year-old man with two years post-oesophagectomy for middle third tumour develops a hoarse voice.

C   A 68-year-old woman with gastric cancer; no metastases on CT scan or EUS.

D   A 45-year-old man with two months' dyspepsia and mild anaemia.

E   A 57-year-old man with jaundice, distal CBD stricture and weight loss.

Question 12. Disorders

Which statements apply to the following conditions?

Options

1   Gastric ulcer.
2   Gastric cancer.
3   Oesophageal cancer.
4   Duodenal ulcer.
5   Gastric MALToma.

Stems

A   Associated with *Helicobacter pylori* infection.

B   Hypogammaglobulinaemia is associated with a 50-fold increased risk.

C   Recurrence is less than 5% after proximal gastric vagotomy.

D   Associated with chronic atrophic gastritis.

E   Following PPI treatment, re-endoscopy and biopsy is recommended.

Pancreatic surgery

Question 13. Acute gallstone pancreatitis

Options

1   ERCP and sphincterotomy.
2   CT scan.
3   MR cholangiogram.
4   Ultrasound.
5   Laparoscopic cholecystectomy and cholangiogram.

Stems

A   A 60-year-old woman 6 days after acute mild gallstone pancreatitis in whom symptoms have resolved.

B   An 84-year-old woman with IHD, 10 days after attack of acute mild gallstone pancreatitis in whom symptoms have resolved.

C   A 45-year-old woman, teetotal, 10 days after attack of acute pancreatitis; no gallstones seen on ultrasound, CBD 7mm.

D   A 55-year-old woman 7 days after acute gallstone pancreatitis with fever and CRP >120 mg/dl.

E   A 63-year-old woman 3 days after acute gallstone pancreatitis, with jaundice and fever.

Question 14. Acute pancreatitis

Options

1   10%.
2   25%.
3   40%.
4   60%.
5   75%.

Stems

A   Proportion of total mortality of acute pancreatitis that occurs in the first week.
B   Overall mortality of acute pancreatitis.
C   Percentage of patients in which there is gallstone aetiology.
D   Percentage of patients classified as mild acute pancreatitis.
E   Overall mortality of severe acute pancreatitis.

Question 15. Complications of acute pancreatitis

These complications of acute pancreatitis occur typically at the following time intervals.

Options

1   24 hours.
2   1 week.
3   2 weeks.
4   4 weeks.
5   6 weeks.

Stems

A   Acute fluid collection.
B   Hypovolaemic shock.
C   Pancreatic abscess.
D   Pancreatic pseudocyst.
E   Splenic artery pseudoaneurysm.

Question 16. Chronic pancreatitis

Associated with forms of chronic pancreatitis.

Options

1 30% of cases of chronic pancreatitis.
2 Autosomal recessive.
3 Pancreatic cyst formation.
4 High risk of pancreatic cancer.
5 Prominent pancreatic calcification.

Stems

A Chronic obstructive pancreatitis.
B Tropical pancreatitis.
C Hereditary pancreatitis.
D Alcohol-induced chronic pancreatitis.
E Idiopathic chronic pancreatitis.

Question 17. Chronic pancreatitis

In the long-term management of chronic pancreatitis.

Options

1 Coeliac plexus block.
2 Distal pancreatectomy.
3 Pancreatojejunostomy.
4 Pancreatic stent.
5 Pancreatic cystgastrostomy.

Stems

A Intractable pain with heavy calcification in the body and tail of the pancreas.
B Pseudocyst 5cm in diameter.
C Pain and dilated pancreatic duct of 15mm.
D Pain and cystic change localised to the tail of the pancreas.
E Intractable pain and onset of diabetes.

Question 18. Risk factors

Options

1   Radiotherapy.
2   *Helicobacter pylori* infection.
3   Smoking.
4   Pancreas divisum.
5   Blood group A.

Stems

A   Gastric cancer.
B   Oesophageal cancer.
C   Pancreatic cancer.
D   Chronic pancreatitis.
E   Acute pancreatitis.

Question 19. Carcinoma of the pancreas

Options

1   2-3%.
2   10%.
3   20%.
4   30%.
5   40%.

Stems

A   Incidence of duodenal obstruction.
B   Resection rate for adenocarcinoma of the body of the pancreas.
C   Resection rate for adenocarcinoma of the head of the pancreas.
D   Overall 5-year survival for all patients with carcinoma of the pancreas.
E   5-year survival post-resection for carcinoma of the pancreas.

Question 20. Endocrine tumours of the pancreas

Options

1   Gastrinoma.
2   VIPoma.
3   PPoma.
4   Insulinoma.
5   Glucagonoma.

Stems

A   Syncope, confusion, obesity.
B   Profuse watery diarrhoea, flushing, hypokalaemia.
C   Abdominal pain, diarrhoea, dysphagia.
D   Asymptomatic.
E   Dermatitis, weight loss, diarrhoea.

Hepatobiliary surgery

Question 21. Investigation

Select the most appropriate investigation(s).

Options

1   HIDA scan.
2   Percutanous transhepatic cholangiogram (PTC).
3   Endoscopic retrograde cholangiogram (ERC).
4   Endoluminal ultrasound (EUS).
5   Magnetic resonance cholangiogram (MRC).

Stems

A   A 33-year-old woman with recent acute pancreatitis, no alcohol history; normal ultrasound, duct 6mm, no jaundice.

B   A 45-year-old man with a previous hepaticojejunostomy 6 years ago for bile duct stricture, develops jaundice.

C   A 76-year-old man with a previous Polya gastrectomy 30 years ago, develops obstructive jaundice.

D   A 68-year-old woman, 4 days post-cholecystectomy, with bile leak.

E   A 24-year-old woman, episodes of recurrent cholangitis; 5cm cystic lesion in porta hepatis on ultrasound.

Question 22. Treatment

Select the most appropriate treatment option.

Options

1   Laparoscopic cholecystectomy and on-table cholangiogram.
2   ERCP and sphincterotomy.
3   CT scan.
4   Percutaneous cholecystostomy.
5   Laparoscopy.

Stems

A   An 88-year-old woman with acute cholecystitis; persistent pyrexia and tender enlarged gall bladder.

B   An 84-year-old woman 10 days post acute gallstone pancreatitis; symptoms resolved and normal LFT.

C   A 34-year-old woman 10 days post acute gallstone pancreatitis; symptoms resolved and normal LFT.

D   A 68-year-old woman 1 month after resolution of gallstone ileus.

E   A 45-year-old woman with severe right upper quadrant pain 4 days after cholecystectomy; normal ultrasound.

Question 23. Disorders

Match the statements.

Options

1   Focal nodular hyperplasia.
2   Primary liver cell carcinoma.
3   Choledochal cyst.
4   Hydatid disease of liver.
5   Colorectal liver metastases.

Stems

A   Increased risk of malignancy.
B   Associated with elevated α-fetoprotein.
C   May cause extrahepatic bile duct obstruction.
D   Associated with haemochromatosis.
E   Associated with chronic hepatitis B infection.

Question 24. Anatomy of Calot's triangle

Options

1   Medial border.
2   Lateral border.
3   Inferior border.
4   Superior border.

Stems

A   Liver.
B   Hartmann's pouch.
C   Cystic duct.
D   Common hepatic duct.
E   Aberrant right hepatic artery from superior mesenteric artery.

Question 25. Liver function tests

Options

1   Prolonged prothrombin time resistant to Vitamin K.
2   Elevated urobilinogen.
3   Elevated unconjugated bilirubin.
4   Elevated aminotransferase level.
5   Positive antimitochrondrial antibody.

Stems

A   Autoimmune haemolytic anaemia.
B   Gilbert's syndrome.
C   End-stage chronic alcoholic hepatitis.
D   Common bile duct stone.
E   Primary biliary cirrhosis.

Question 26. Diagnosis

Select the most likely diagnosis.

Options

1   Hepatic abscess.
2   Common bile duct stricture.
3   Liver adenoma.
4   Ascending cholangitis.
5   Sclerosing cholangitis.

Stems

A   A 64-year-old man with right upper quadrant pain, jaundice and
     pyrexia of 38.5.
B   A 33-year-old woman, 10 years salazopyrine treatment for
     diarrhoea and bleeding, develops jaundice.
C   An 84-year-old man, previous history of diverticular disease,
     develops right upper quadrant pain and swinging pyrexia of 37.5.
D   A 64-year-old woman, 3-month history of back pain and weight
     loss, develops jaundice.
E   A 38-year-old woman, 15 years of oral contraceptive use,
     develops acute severe right upper quadrant pain and hypotension.

Question 27. Unresectable carcinomas

For the following unresectable carcinomas.

Options

1 Gemcitabine.
2 Radiotherapy.
3 5-Fluorouracil.
4 Streptozotocin.
5 Tamoxifen.

Stems

A Oesophageal cancer.
B Gastric cancer.
C Pancreatic cancer.
D Metastatic gastrinoma.
E Colorectal liver metastases.

Question 28. Gallstone disease

Options

1 Conservative.
2 ERCP and stent.
3 Laparoscopic cholecystectomy.
4 Exploration common bile duct and T-tube.
5 Exploration common bile duct and choledochoduodenostomy.

Stems

A A 45-year-old man found to have incidental porcelain gall bladder on x-ray.
B A 68-year-old man with stone impacted in the common bile duct, unable to be removed at ERCP.
C A 38-year-old woman found to have incidental gallstones on ultrasound requested for pelvic symptoms.
D A 94-year-old woman with acute cholecystitis.
E A 44-year-old man with Mirizzi syndrome.

Answer 1   A5, B1, (or 4), C3, D4, E2

High-grade dysplasia is an indication for oesophagectomy, but in this example the patient's comorbidity precludes it. For patients B and D the aim of management is symptom control. Neoadjuvant chemotherapy is generally advocated for T3 or node-positive tumours.

Answer 2   A1, B2, C2, D3, E none

Refer to BSG guidelines (www.bsg.org.uk) for investigation of dyspepsia. Failure to respond to antacids (patient E) is difficult. Further investigation is warranted - the lack of response to antacids suggests another cause such as biliary colic. Ultrasound would be advised.

Answer 3   A4, B3, C2, D1, E5

Answer 4   A3, B4, C2 & 1, D4, E1

Dysmotility is not a contraindication to anti-reflux surgery; studies have not shown an increased incidence of postoperative dysphagia. Normal 24-hour acid exposure is pH <4 for <4% of the study duration. Patient E shows only modest reflux and would be best managed with medical therapy.

Answer 5   A3, B1, C1, (3), D4, E2, 5, (1, 3).

Ménétriere's disease leads to enormous gastric protein loss. Para-oesophageal hernia may lead to a 'riding' ulcer and chronic Fe-deficiency anaemia. Gastric cancer is frequently associated with chronic blood loss and low serum protein if advanced. Post-gastrectomy B_{12} supplements are required: fat malabsorption may lead to Vitamin D deficiency. Fe-deficiency and low serum albumin only occur if dietary intake is inadequate.

Answer 6   A1, (or 3), B4, C2, (or 1), D2, (or 4), E none

Guidelines for the management of acute upper GI bleeding can be found at www.bsg.org.uk. Initial control of variceal bleeding should be by injection sclerotherapy or rubber-band ligation. Re-bleed from a gastric ulcer is an indication for surgery. Initial therapy for a duodenal ulcer is by heater probe or injection sclerotherapy; laser therapy is no longer used. Dieulafoy's lesions often require surgery.

Answer 7   A5, B1, C2, D1, E4

Overall 5-year survival for resected oesophageal cancer (curative resection, all stages) is 25%; for resected gastric cancer, 50%.

Answer 8   A5, B3, C2, D4, E1

Answer 9   A3, B1, C4, D4, E2

In the absence of metastases and if the patient is fit, resection is the most effective palliation for obstructing or bleeding gastric cancer. Total gastrectomy is required for middle and proximal third tumours with D2 node dissection; 80% partial gastrectomy for distal third tumours. No survival advantage is conferred by the addition of splenectomy or pancreatectomy.

Answer 10   A4, B3, C1, D2, E5

Answer 11   A5, (4), B1, C2, D4, E1 & 3

Patient A suggests a pharyngeal pouch. Barium swallow is the preferred first-line investigation though endoscopy may be performed as long as this diagnosis is kept in mind. Staging laparoscopy should be performed prior to resection for all gastric and lower third oesophageal tumours. Patient E suggests carcinoma of the pancreas. EUS provides the most accurate local staging information; a CT scan detects distant metastases.

Answer 12   A1, 4 & 5, B2, C none, D2, E1

Duodenal ulcer, gastric cancer and gastric MALToma are all associated with HP infection. Recurrence of duodenal ulcer is >10% 5 years after proximal vagotomy.

Answer 13   A5, (1), B1, C4, (3), D2, E1

Refer to BSG guidelines for the management of acute pancreatitis (www.bsg.org.uk). Stone clearance, either by ERCP or cholecystectomy, is recommended as soon as possible after acute gallstone pancreatitis. In the elderly and unfit, sphincterotomy may be definitive therapy. In fit, young patients, cholecystectomy with a cholangiogram showing the duct is clear prevents the need for ERCP. Repeat ultrasound is helpful in patient C as gallstones may be missed on the original scan due to overlying bowel gas. MRC is an alternative, but CBD stones have usually passed.

Answer 14   A4, B1, C3, D5, E2

Answer 15   A2, (3), B1, C4, D5, (4), E5 (4)

Peripancreatic fluid is defined as an acute fluid collection before 4 weeks; pancreatic pseudocyst after this time.

Answer 16   A3, B5, C4 & 5, D5, E1

Heavy pancreatic calcification is seen in tropical and hereditary pancreatitis. Alcohol is the commonest cause of chronic pancreatitis (>50%) followed by idiopathic (30%). Hereditary pancreatitis is autosomal dominant and associated with a high risk of pancreatic cancer.

Answer 17   A2, B none, C3, (4), D2, E none

Coeliac plexus block provides poor long-term pain relief in chronic pancreatitis. Resection may be helpful for disease localised to one section of the pancreas. Surgery is not recommended for pseudocysts <6cm. Drainage is often helpful for pain secondary to pancreatic obstruction: operative drainage is preferred to a stent.

Answer 18   A2, 3 & 5, B3, C3, D4, E1

Answer 19   A3, B1, C3, D1, E2

Answer 20   A4, B2, C1, D3, E5

Answer 21   A4, (5), B1, (2), C2, D3, E5, (3)

EUS is sensitive at detecting microcalculi in patient A. An HIDA scan is useful at detecting problems at a bilio-enteric anastomosis by demonstrating delay of isotope excretion, although PTC may be required for therapeutic procedures. After Polya gastrectomy, access to the bile duct by ERC is not usually possible. ERC is the first-line investigation for bile leak and allows stent placement.

Answer 22   A4, B2, C1, D none, E5

For acute cholecystitis, early cholecystectomy is preferred; for the elderly or unfit, percutaneous cholecystostomy is a good alternative. Similarly, early cholecystectomy is recommended for acute gallstone pancreatitis; in the elderly, endoscopic sphincterotomy is appropriate. Cholecystectomy is not required after gallstone ileus. Although ultrasound is normal in patient E, the symptoms and signs are severe and urgent laparoscopy is indicated.

Answer 23   A3, B2, C4 & 5, D2, E2.

Extrahepatic bile duct obstruction may be caused by rupture of a hydatid into the biliary tree and with malignant porta hepatis nodes in colorectal cancer.

Answer 24   A4, B none, C3, D1, E1.

Calot's triangle is bounded superiorly by the liver, inferiorly by the cystic duct and medially by the common hepatic duct. In 15% of people an aberrant right hepatic artery runs alongside the common hepatic duct.

Answer 25 A3, B3, C1 & 4, D none, E5.

Answer 26 A4, B5, C1, D2, E3.

In patient A this represents Charcot's triad. Sclerosing cholangitis is strongly associated with ulcerative colitis. Patient D is very suggestive of pancreatic cancer causing biliary obstruction. Liver adenoma is associated with long-term contraceptive pill use and may present with acute rupture, haemorrhage and collapse.

Answer 27 A2, B none, C1, D4, E3.

Radiotherapy offers good palliation for dysphagia in oesophageal cancer. Gemcitabine is approved by the National Institute for Clinical Excellence (NICE) for unresectable pancreatic cancer. A clinical response has been reported with streptozotocin in malignant gastrinoma. 5-fluorouracil is the most effective agent for colorectal cancer.

Answer 28 A3, B5, (4 or 2), C1, D1, E2.

Porcelain gallbladder is associated with an increased risk of gallbladder cancer. For patient B the preferred management is exploration of the bile duct with T-tube drainage or choledochoduodenostomy. Stent placement is a temporary measure. Asymptomatic gallstones do not require treatment. A biliary stent is used to relieve jaundice in Mirizzi syndrome and allows acute inflammation to resolve before proceeding to subtotal cholecystectomy.

Chapter 10

Colorectal surgery

Aileen McKinley, FRCS
Consultant Surgeon, Aberdeen Royal Infirmary, Aberdeen, UK
Terry O'Kelly, MD FRCS
Consultant Surgeon, Aberdeen Royal Infirmary, Aberdeen, UK

For all questions each option may be used once, more than once or not at all.

Question 1. Symptoms of benign colorectal disease

From each of the clinical scenarios, select the most likely diagnosis from the options listed.

Options

1   Anal fissure.
2   Perianal abscess.
3   Haemorrhoids.
4   Ulcerative colitis.
5   Pilonidal abscess.
6   Anal fistula.
7   Proctalgia fugax.

Stems

A   30-year-old female presenting with diarrhoea 10 times per day, with blood mixed with stool.

B   20-year-old male complaining of acute pain PR and fresh bleeding on opening bowels.

C   55-year-old male emergency admission with severe pain on the left buttock.

D   35-year-old female with a history of intermittent painless bleeding PR, pruritis ani and tissue prolapse.

E   25-year-old male with a painful, discharging lump in the natal cleft.

F   27-year-old male complains of intermittent, spasmodic anorectal pain, usually precipitated by intercourse.

Question 2. Colorectal cancer surgery

Choose the most suitable surgical procedure for resection of the following cancers.

Options

1   Extended right hemicolectomy.
2   Anterior resection.
3   Left hemicolectomy.
4   Abdominoperineal resection.
5   Right hemicolectomy.

Stems

A   Tumour in the upper third of rectum.
B   Tumour in the mid-transverse colon.
C   Tumour in the caecum.
D   Tumour in the descending colon.
E   Tumour in the lower rectum, involving the anal sphincter complex.

Question 3. Symptoms of colorectal disease

Choose the most common presenting feature for each of the conditions below.

Options

1   Recurrent, intermittent left-sided abdominal pain over the last few years.
2   Pneumaturia.
3   Anaemia.
4   Altered bowel habit and PR bleeding.
5   Tenesmus.
6   Vomiting.

Stems

A   Tumour in the lower rectum.
B   Caecal cancer.
C   Colo-vesical fistula.
D   Diverticular disease.
E   Sigmoid cancer.

Question 4. Colorectal cancer screening

The following asymptomatic patients have asked you for advice regarding colorectal cancer (CRC) screening on the basis of their family history. Choose the most suitable advice for each of them. You may select more than one option for each case if appropriate.

Options

1   Colonoscopy.
2   Referral to the clinical genetic service regarding gene testing.
3   Discuss gynaecological screening for endometrial and ovarian cancer.
4   Reassurance and advice on healthy eating only.
5   Barium enema and flexible sigmoidoscopy.

Stems

A   65-year-old female, father died of colorectal cancer aged 80.

B   40-year-old male, mother died of colorectal cancer aged 45 years, one maternal uncle diagnosed with CRC aged 42, and maternal grandmother died of CRC aged 50.

C   39-year-old male, mother diagnosed with CRC aged 44.

D   54-year-old female with strong family history of diverticular disease in three first degree relatives under 50 years of age.

E   39-year-old female, mother diagnosed with CRC aged 49, one maternal aunt with endometrial cancer aged 45, and maternal grandfather diagnosed with CRC aged 55 years.

Question 5. Colorectal cancer and polyp surveillance

Choose the most suitable follow-up protocol for the following patients.

Options

1   No further colonic investigation required.
2   Repeat colonoscopy in 3-6 months.
3   Repeat colonoscopy in 3-5 years.
4   Barium enema and flexible sigmoidoscopy.
5   CT colonography / virtual colonoscopy.

Stems

A   Large sessile polyp, removed piecemeal - histology benign.

B   Rectal polyp biopsied at colonoscopy, performed to investigate altered bowel habit - histology showed metaplasia only.

C   Anterior resection for CRC 5 years ago. Check colonoscopy this year was completely clear.

D   Patient with ulcerative colitis (for 15 years), colonic biopsy showed high-grade dysplasia and patient decided to proceed to total proctocolectomy and ileostomy.

E   Single large sigmoid polyp (>2cm) removed at colonoscopy - histology showed a tubulovillous adenoma with low-grade dysplasia and excision appears complete.

Question 6. Clinico-pathological features of Inflammatory Bowel Disease (IBD)

Choose the features that are consistent with the conditions below. You may select more than one option for each stem if appropriate.

Options

1   Inflammation affects the full thickness of the bowel wall.
2   Inflammation affects the mucosal and submucosal layers of the bowel wall only.
3   May affect the oesophagus.
4   Fistulae are a common complication.
5   Granulomata may be seen on histological examination.
6   The rectum is almost always involved.

Stems

A   Crohn's disease.
B   Ulcerative colitis.

Question 7. Fluid and electrolyte balance

In order to calculate postoperative fluid replacement regimes correctly, it is important to know the normal daily adult requirements and losses. Choose the figures that are appropriate for the stems below.

Options

1   5-10.
2   40-50.
3   80-100.
4   120-130.
5   140-150.

Stems

A   Normal daily potassium requirement (mmol).
B   Normal daily sodium requirement (mmol).
C   Potassium concentration in gastric secretion (mmol/l).
D   Daily urinary sodium loss (mmol).
E   Daily urinary potassium loss (mmol).

Question 8. Pelvic nerve function

Select the appropriate nerve supply for the following functions.

Options

1   L5.
2   Pudendal nerve (S2-4).
3   Sympathetic via hypogastric nerves (T10-L2).
4   Somatic via the genitofemoral nerve.
5   Enteric recto-anal innervation.
6   Ilioinguinal nerve (L1).

Stems

A   Contraction of the bladder neck.
B   Contraction of the pelvic floor (levator ani).
C   Relaxation of the internal anal sphincter.
D   External anal sphincter contraction.

Question 9. Grading of haemorrhoids

From the information given for the following patients, classify the grade of haemorrhoids described.

Options

1   First degree.
2   Second degree.

3   Third degree.
4   Fourth degree.

Stems

A   Patient describes haemorrhoids that prolapse after defecation and require manual reduction.
B   Haemorrhoids only evident above the dentate line on proctoscopy.
C   Small haemorrhoids with no prolapse and occasional bleeding.
D   Patient describes intermittent prolapse of haemorrhoids that reduce spontaneously.
E   Patient presents with irreducible prolapsed haemorrhoids.

Question 10. Management of haemorrhoids

Select one suitable management strategy for each of the following patients. In each case, serious underlying pathology has been excluded.

Options

1   Rubber band ligation.
2   Stapled haemorrhoidopexy.
3   Surgical haemorrhoidectomy.
4   Conservative measures: high fibre diet, topical preparations, bulk laxatives.

Stems

A   Circumferential third degree haemorrhoids.
B   Minor intermittent bleeding only from first degree haemorrhoids.
C   Large external haemorrhoids with troublesome anal canal bleeding.
D   Prolapsed irreducible haemorrhoids.
E   Single prolapsing, bleeding haemorrhoid.

Question 11. Risk of venous thromboembolism (VTE) in colorectal surgery

Estimate the risk of venous thromboembolism after the following procedures for colorectal disease.

Options

1   No risk.
2   Low risk.
3   Moderate risk.
4   High risk.

Stems

A   Anterior resection for rectal cancer in a 65-year-old man.
B   EUA for recurrent fissure-in-ano in a 35-year-old man.
C   EUA for a low rectal fistula in a 30-year-old female with a history of previous DVT in pregnancy.
D   Colonoscopy.
E   Reversal of ileostomy in a 40-year-old man with a body mass index (BMI) of 36.

Question 12. Anticoagulation in colorectal surgery

Which one of the following means of anticoagulation would you use initially for the patients described?

Options

1   Low molecular weight heparin - prophylaxis dose.
2   Low molecular weight heparin - treatment dose.
3   Unfractionated heparin infusion.
4   Warfarin.
5   Caval filter placement.

Stems

A   Patient with an artificial (metal) heart valve 1 day after a difficult low anterior resection.

B   Patient with newly diagnosed femoral DVT, 5 days after sigmoid colectomy.

C   Pre-operative DVT prophylaxis for patient at high-risk of venous thrombosis before abdominoperineal resection.

D   Patient having recurrent pulmonary emboli postoperatively, after low anterior resection, despite adequate medical therapy.

E   Treatment for patient B (above) with postoperative femoral DVT, now 10 days after surgery and almost ready for discharge home.

Question 13. The pharmacological properties of laxative preparations

Indicate the type of preparation for each laxative preparation.

Options

1   Bulk forming agent.
2   Stool softener.
3   Stimulant laxative.
4   Osmotic laxative.

Stems

A   Lactulose.
B   Senna.
C   Arachis oil enema.
D   Phosphate enema.
E   Fybogel (ispaghula husk).
F   Bran.

Question 14. Therapeutic options in ulcerative colitis (UC)

Choose the most appropriate initial therapy for each of these patients with UC.

Options

1   Immodium.
2   Mesalazine.
3   Mebeverine.
4   Corticosteroids.
5   Surgery.

Stems

A   Emergency admission with a new diagnosis of UC and toxic dilation of the colon on x-ray, which has developed despite adequate medical therapy.

B   Frequent (x 6 per day) loose, bloody stool.

C   Relapse of disease despite an adequate course of aminosalicylate.

D   High-grade dysplasia on colonic biopsy in a patient with a 15-year history of active colitis.

Question 15. Management of anal fissure

Select the most suitable treatment for each of these patients with anal fissure.

Options

1   Conservative measures - high fibre diet and laxatives as required.
2   Topical 0.2% GTN ointment.
3   Lateral sphincterotomy.
4   Anal stretch.
5   EUA +/- biopsy.
6   Injection of botulinum toxin.

Stems

A   30-year-old female with 6 weeks of pain on defecation, with bright red bleeding.

B   35-year-old male who returns to the clinic with persistent pain after 3 months of nitrate therapy.

C   59-year-old admitted as an emergency with intense anal pain.

D   40-year-old attending clinic for review; now asymptomatic with healed anal fissure.

E   55-year-old man who returns to clinic with persistent pain and unable to tolerate even low doses of nitrate due to headaches.

Question 16. Colorectal cancer - Dukes' staging

Select the correct Dukes' stage from the information provided.

Options

1   Dukes' stage A.

2   Dukes' stage B.

3   Dukes' stage C1.

4   Dukes' stage C2.

Stems

A   Tumour invades through to the serosa and involves the adjacent bladder wall. 17 lymph nodes examined were all free from tumour.

B   Tumour is confined to the mucosa and all lymph nodes examined are free from disease.

C   Tumour is confined to the mucosa; 4 out of 11 lymph nodes are positive for tumour.

D   Tumour infiltrates the muscularis mucosa; 8 out of 10 lymph nodes have tumour present (including the apical node).

E   Tumour invades the muscularis mucosa; all lymph nodes are clear.

Question 17. Colorectal cancer - TNM staging

Select the correct TNM stage from the information provided.

Options

1	T2 N1 M0.
2	T3 N2 M0.
3	T4 N1 M0.
4	T1 N0 M0.
5	T3 N1 M1.
6	T3 N2 M1.
7	T2 N2 M1.

Stems

A Tumour invades through serosa into bladder; 3 out of 16 lymph nodes positive for tumour.

B Tumour invades muscularis propria; metastases evident in 3 out of 12 lymph nodes examined.

C Tumour invades submucosa; no lymph node metastases seen.

D Tumour invades into the subserosa; metastases evident in 6 out of 12 lymph nodes.

E Tumour invades through into the subserosa; 2 out of 8 lymph nodes positive; liver metastases on ultrasound scan.

Question 18. Histology

What histological findings would you expect on examination of the following specimens?

Options

1	Squamous cell carcinoma.
2	Adenocarcinoma.
3	Dysplasia.
4	Hamartoma.
5	Carcinoid tumour.

Stems

A   Colonic polyp in patient with Peutz-Jegher's syndrome.
B   Anal carcinoma.
C   Tumour of the appendix.
D   Large (>1cm) tubulovillous adenoma.
E   Rectal carcinoma.

Question 19. Anatomy - lymphatic drainage

Select the initial site of lymphatic drainage for the stems below.

Options

1   Superficial inguinal lymph nodes.
2   Internal iliac lymph nodes.
3   Para-aortic nodes.
4   Inferior mesenteric lymph nodes.
5   Supraclavicular nodes.

Stems

A   Lower vagina and labia.
B   Anus, below the dentate line.
C   Anus, above the dentate line.
D   Skin of the buttock.
E   Sigmoid colon.

Question 20. Anatomy - arterial supply

Select the correct arterial blood supply for the stems below.

Options

1   Superior mesenteric artery.
2   Inferior rectal artery.
3   Superior rectal artery.
4   Middle colic artery.
5   Ileocolic artery.
6   Inferior mesenteric artery.

Stems

A   The upper rectum is supplied principally by the...
B   The caecum is supplied by the ...
C   The hindgut structures are supplied by the ...
D   The proximal transverse colon is supplied by the ...
E   The appendix is supplied by a branch of the ...

Question 21. Rectal examination

Select the correct figure for each of the stems below.

Options

1   2cm.
2   4cm.
3   10cm.
4   12cm.
5   20cm.

Stems

A   From the anal verge, the average adult finger can examine the rectum to a height of ...
B   The average length of the rectum is ...

C   From the anal verge, the rigid sigmoidoscope can give a view up to approximately ...

D   The average length of the anal canal in adults is ...

Question 22. Definitions in colorectal surgery

Select the correct definition for the stems below.

Options

1   An abnormal communication between two epithelial surfaces.
2   Collection of fluid in a sac lined by endo- or epithelium.
3   Linear breach in the squamous epithelium.
4   Breach in an epithelial surface.
5   Blind epithelial tract extending onto skin.

Stems

A   Fissure.
B   Fistula.
C   Sinus.
D   Ulcer.
E   Cyst.

Question 23. Complications after major colorectal surgery

Select the most common timescale for development of the complications below.

Options

1   Intra-operative.
2   1 day.
3   3 days.
4   5 days.
5   7 days.

Stems

A   Pulmonary embolism.
B   Anastomotic leak.
C   Pulmonary atelectasis
D   Major bleeding.
E   DVT.

Question 24. Embryology

Select the correct embryological origin for the stems below.

Options

1   Foregut.
2   Midgut.
3   Hindgut.
4   Urachus.
5   Vitello-intestinal duct.
6   Umbilical artery.

Stems

A   The rectum.
B   Proximal third of the transverse colon.
C   Meckels diverticulum.
D   Splenic flexure.
E   Appendix.

Question 25. Stoma formation

Select the correct type of stoma appropriate for each of the stems below.

Options

1   Hartmann's.
2   Permanent end colostomy.

3   Caecostomy.
4   Percutaneous gastrostomy (PEG).
5   Loop ileostomy.
6   Spout ileostomy.

Stems

A   Total colectomy for colonic Crohn's disease.
B   Low anterior resection with formation of colon pouch in a patient after pre-operative radiotherapy.
C   Abdominoperineal resection.
D   Restorative proctocolectomy.
E   Perforated diverticular disease.

Question 26. Presenting features of diverticular disease

Select the correct diagnosis for each of the clinical scenarios in the stems below.

Options

1   Acute diverticulitis.
2   Diverticular disease.
3   Acute phlegmonous diverticulitis.
4   Diverticular fistula.
5   Diverticular free perforation.

Stems

A   Emergency presentation with left lower quadrant pain, fever, malaise and a palpable mass in the left iliac fossa (LIF).
B   Patient attends the outpatient clinic with a history of recurrent urinary tract infection and a 'bubbling' sensation on passing urine.
C   Patient with previous self-limiting episodes of intermittent LIF pain and diarrhoea presents as an emergency with similar symptoms and mild systemic upset.

D   Patient presents as an emergency moribund with a rigid abdomen on examination.

E   Finding of scattered sigmoid diverticula on a barium enema performed to investigate altered bowel habit.

Question 27. Management of diverticular disease

Select the most suitable management strategy for each of the cases described in the stems below.

Options

1   Sigmoid colectomy and primary anastomosis.
2   Hartmann's resection.
3   Percutaneous drainage of abscess under USS or CT control.
4   Sigmoid colectomy and primary anastomosis with covering loop ileostomy.
5   Colostomy only.
6   Conservative management: high fibre and fluid intake.

Stems

A   A fit 70-year-old man with two previous admissions with significant lower GI haemorrhage presents with a third acute bleed. Selective mesenteric angiography shows active bleeding from the lower sigmoid colon.

B   An obese 75-year-old female presents as an emergency, moribund, with a rigid abdomen on examination. At laparotomy, perforated diverticular disease is found.

C   Asymptomatic patient with diverticular disease (found incidentally at a screening colonoscopy for a strong family history of CRC).

D   Patient is scheduled for elective surgery for troublesome, recurrent bouts of acute diverticulitis. Currently, he is pain-free with no evidence of systemic upset.

E   An 80-year-old man with recent history of myocardial infarction (6 weeks ago) and known diverticular disease is admitted from a nursing home with a fluctuating fever, and a tender LIF mass - the rest of the abdomen is soft.

Question 28. Intestinal obstruction

Select the most likely operative procedure required for each of the stems below.

Options

1 Colonic stenting.
2 Extended right hemicolectomy.
3 Subtotal colectomy and ileorectal anastomosis.
4 Right hemicolectomy.
5 Colonoscopic decompression.
6 Adhesiolysis.

Stems

A 85-year-old male with gross abdominal distension and mild abdominal discomfort 5 days after surgery for a fractured neck of femur. Bowel sounds are quiet.

B 85-year-old demented male presents for a second time in 18 months with a sigmoid volvulus.

C 23-year-old male with colicky central abdominal pain and dilated small bowel loops on plain abdominal x-ray. Previous surgical history includes appendicectomy aged 13, and orchidopexy aged 4 years.

D 89-year-old with significant infective exacerbation of severe emphysema presents with an obstructing sigmoid carcinoma.

E 70-year-old male with an obstructing carcinoma in the mid-transverse colon.

Question 29. PR bleeding

Select the most likely cause of bleeding for each of the stems below.

Options

1   Ischaemic colitis.
2   Angiodysplasia.
3   Diverticular disease.
4   Anal fissure.
5   Caecal carcinoma.
6   Haemorrhoids.

Stems

A   65-year-old female attends for investigation with a 3-month history of lethargy and weight loss. Her haemoglobin is 80g/dl and three stool FOB samples are positive.

B   35-year-old female (para 2+0) with painless rectal bleeding that occurs after defecation intermittently. Fresh blood is usually only seen on the paper.

C   70-year-old male with severe angina and no history of bowel problems presents as an emergency with acute onset left-sided abdominal pain and profuse bloody diarrhoea. Abdominal x-ray shows no evidence of obstruction of perforation.

D   75-year-old female with recurrent iron-deficiency anaemia. Extensive investigations of the GI tract have not identified any source of blood loss.

Question 30. Abdominal wall hernias

Options

1   Sliding hernia.
2   Littre's hernia.
3   Richter's hernia.
4   Maydl's hernia.
5   Spigelian hernia.

Stems

A   In this type of hernia, a W-loop of small bowel may become strangulated within the hernial sac.
B   If only part of the circumference of the bowel wall is involved, the hernia is called a ...
C   Bowel herniating through the lateral border of the rectus sheath is known as a ...
D   One wall of the hernial sac is formed by a viscus (eg. bladder or caecum) which forms part of the hernia, but is outside the cavity of the peritoneal sac.
E   A strangulated Meckel's diverticulum is contained in a ...

Answer 1   A4, B1, C2, D3, E5, F7

Common causes of bloody diarrhoea in a young patient include acute gastroenteritis (such as Campylobacter or Salmonella infection) and inflammatory bowel disease (ulcerative colitis and Crohn's disease). In the acute situation it is important to obtain stools for culture to exclude an infectious cause.

Anal fissure is a common cause of anal pain and bleeding. In the acute situation, the patient will often not be able to tolerate examination in the clinic. Most patients present with a primary fissure, but secondary fissures can also be caused by Crohn's disease, trauma, infection and malignancy.

Haemorrhoids most commonly present with bleeding on defecation and intermittent prolapse. Additional symptoms may include discomfort, itching, swelling and minor soiling. Acute severe pain suggests the development of a complication such as irreducible prolapse and thrombosis. Recurrent pain with defecation is uncommon with haemorrhoids and suggests the presence of a fissure-in-ano.

Acute pilonidal abscess typically presents with a painful lump in the upper natal cleft. There are often visible pits in the midline overlying the swelling. Pilonidal disease occurs more commonly in post-pubertal males and symptoms are uncommon beyond the fourth decade. Pilonidal abscesses can be usually differentiated from perianal abscesses by their position in the natal cleft, although perianal pilonidal disease can occur from entrapment of hair in the scar after anal surgery.

Proctalgia fugax is a non-specific symptom of transient shooting pain in the rectum. It is rarely associated with significant disease.

Answer 2   A2, B1, C5, D3, E4

Colonic resections for cancer are performed to remove any tumour together with draining lymph nodes. If a low rectal cancer involves the anal sphincter complex, then adequate tumour clearance may only be obtained by removing the anus in an abdominoperineal resection.

Bowel resections are determined by the arterial blood supply to the colon. Tumours in the mid-transverse colon to the splenic flexure region are best dealt with by extended right hemicolectomy due to the arterial supply. The blood supply at the splenic flexure usually relies on an anastomosis between the middle and left colic arteries. However, this can be variable. In 6% there is no left colic artery and the blood supply then depends on the middle colic artery. In 22% there is no middle colic artery and the blood supply then comes from both right and left colic arteries. Since the lymphatic drainage follows the arterial supply, it would seem sensible to ligate the right, middle and left colic arteries, making an extended right hemicolectomy necessary.

Answer 3   A5, (or 4), B3, C2, D1, E4

Tenesmus is an uncomfortable desire to defecate when there is no stool present in the rectum. It can be caused by a rectal tumour or by rectal inflammation.

The contents of the caecum and ascending colon are fluid in consistency and therefore, altered bowel habit and obstruction tend to be late features. Instead, caecal malignancies often present with microcytic, hypochromic anaemia due to chronic occult blood loss, or with right iliac fossa discomfort and a palpable mass.

Pneumaturia (bubbling on micturition) is a sign of a fistula between the gut and bladder. Diverticular disease is the most common cause of a colovesical fistula. Crohn's disease, previous pelvic radiotherapy and pelvic malignancy may also cause formation of a colovesical fistula.

Answer 4   A4, B1 & 2, C1, D4, E1, 2 & 3

Further details on prevention and screening can be found in the SIGN Guidelines for Management of Colorectal Cancer (Guideline Number 67) at www.sign.ac.uk. The investigation of choice for screening on the basis of a strongly positive family history is colonoscopy, since therapeutic polypectomy can be performed at the same examination if polyps are found. If colonoscopy is not complete, then barium enema should be performed.

Patients B and E fulfil the Amsterdam criteria for hereditary non-polyposis colorectal cancer (HNPCC):

(a)   At least three relatives with an HNPCC-associated cancer (colorectal cancer, endometrial, small bowel, ureter or renal pelvis), one of whom should be a first degree relative of the other two.
(b)   At least one case must be diagnosed before the age of 50 years.
(c)   Cases must be present over at least two consecutive generations.
(d)   FAP is excluded.

Families fulfilling the Amsterdam criteria are high-risk for the development of colorectal cancer and therefore, should be offered evaluation and counselling by a clinical geneticist regarding gene testing.

Answer 5   A2, B1, C3, D1, E3

Protocols for colorectal cancer and polyp surveillance can be found on the British Society of Gastroenterology website (www.bsg.org.uk) and are published in *Gut* 2002, volume 51, Supplement V.

CT colonography is not a recognised method for colon surveillance. The high radiation dose associated with CT examinations is not acceptable for recurrent assessment.

Colon surveillance is performed to detect and remove pre-malignant polyps. Barium enema is not the first choice for surveillance, since small polyps may be missed. Also, if polyps are detected at barium enema examination, a further procedure is then required for removal.

Answer 6   A1, 3, 4 & 5, B2 & 6

Crohn's disease is a transmural chronic inflammatory process that can affect any part of the gastrointestinal tract, from mouth to anus. Non-caseating giant cell granulomata are a characteristic histological feature of Crohn's disease, but are only found in 60-70% of cases. Fistula formation occurs in up to 20% of patients with Crohn's disease.

Ulcerative colitis is a disease of the large bowel, with inflammation limited to the mucosa and submucosa. Both Crohn's disease and ulcerative colitis may be associated with extra-intestinal manifestations such as arthropathy, pyoderma gangrenosum and erythema nodosum.

Answer 7   A3, B5, C1, D5, E3

Answer 8   A3, B2, C5, D2

Pelvic sympathetic fibres from the hypogastic plexus are motor to the visceral (smooth) muscle sphincters of the bladder and anal canal. The internal anal sphincter has an intrinsic nerve supply from the myenteric plexus in addition to its extrinsic autonomic supply.

The somatic inferior rectal branches of the pudendal nerve supply the skeletal muscle of the external anal sphincter. The pudendal nerve also supplies the muscles of the perineum and is sensory to the external genitalia.

Answer 9   A3, B1, C1, D2, E4

The clinical grading of haemorrhoids by 'degrees' categorises those that cause bleeding only (first degree), those that prolapse and reduce spontaneously (second degree), those that prolapse and require reduction (third degree), and finally those that prolapse and are not reducible (fourth degree). It is often best, however, to describe the clinical features present since this avoids misinterpretation.

Answer 10   A2 or 3, B4, C3, D3, E1

Many patients with haemorrhoids will require no active treatment. Exclusion of underlying serious pathology, explanation of the problem and advice on conservative measures are often all that is necessary.

Rubber band ligation is most suitable for troublesome bleeding in the absence of a significant external component. Surgery is necessary to deal with symptomatic external haemorrhoids.

Stapled haemorrhoidopexy is a relatively new technique used to treat circumferential and prolapsing haemorrhoids. Results on the long-term efficacy of the procedure are not yet available.

Answer 11   A4, B2, C4, D2, E3

The risk of VTE is influenced by a long list of patient and procedure-related factors - the risk is never absolutely zero. To reduce the potential complication of VTE, it is good practice to encourage loss of excess weight prior to non-urgent elective procedures. Female patients taking the oral contraceptive pill should be counselled regarding the balance of risks and benefits of stopping these preparations before elective surgery.

During surgery the use of intermittent pneumatic compression boots (eg. Flowtron) reduces the incidence of DVT. It is important to prescribe prophylactic low molecular weight heparin and graduated compression (TED) stockings for the period when the patient is less mobile, and to encourage early mobilisation in the postoperative period.

Further details on the prevention of VTE can be found in the SIGN Guidelines for Prophylaxis of Venous Thromboembolism (Guideline Number 62) at www.sign.ac.uk.

Answer 12   A3, B2, C1, D5, E4

Prophylactic measures for the prevention of venous thromboembolism are as described in the notes on Question 11.

In the peri-operative period after major surgery there is a significant risk of bleeding if treatment doses of anticoagulation are administered. The balance of risk and benefit must be assessed for each individual case. If anticoagulation is essential, then an intravenous infusion of unfractionated heparin is preferable since the effects of this are rapidly reversed on stopping the infusion. Unfractionated heparin has a short half-life and the effects of the drug can also be reversed using protamine.

A newly diagnosed DVT or PE should initially be treated with some form of heparin to prevent clot propagation. If there is no risk of exacerbating surgical bleeding, then the use of treatment doses of LMWH is more convenient since monitoring of blood levels is not required.

Once a newly diagnosed DVT or PE has been treated with heparin initially, then warfarin may be commenced. Warfarin antagonises the effects of vitamin K and takes 48 to 72 hours to become fully effective. There should therefore be an overlap in heparin and warfarin therapy, until the warfarin level becomes therapeutic. If there is evidence of ongoing PE despite adequate medical therapy, then placement of a vena caval filter should be considered.

Answer 13   A4, B3, C2, D4, E1, F1

Bulk forming laxatives (such as Fybogel) relieve constipation by increasing the faecal mass which then stimulates peristalsis. A similar effect is achieved by increasing dietary fibre intake. Adequate fluid intake is important with the use of fibre and bulk laxatives in constipation.

Stimulant laxatives (bisacodyl, senna, docusate sodium) increase intestinal motility and may cause intestinal cramps. These drugs should be avoided in the presence of intestinal obstruction.

Osmotic laxatives (lactulose, phosphate enema) exert their effect by increasing the amount of water in the large bowel.

See the British National Formulary (www.BNF.org) for further reading.

Answer 14   A5, B2, C4, D5

The initial management of ulcerative colitis depends on the degree of severity and the extent of the disease at presentation. Treatment is medical in most cases. Steroids are used to induce remission while 5-aminosalicylate preparations (eg. mesalazine) are used to maintain remission once it has been achieved.

A small group of patients present with severe acute colitis and, despite maximal medical therapy, toxic dilation of the colon develops. These cases require urgent surgery.

Patients with long-standing colitis are at increased risk of colorectal cancer. The presence of low- or high-grade dysplasia on biopsy is an indication for resection of the colon.

Answer 15   A2, B3, C5, D1, E3

Most acute fissures heal spontaneously. Conservative measures may aid this by softening stools and relieving pain. In most cases, a trial of medical therapy is appropriate before proceeding to surgical intervention.

Medical treatments include glyceryl trinitrate ointment (0.2%), which acts to reduce anal pressure and achieves healing in 50-70% of fissures.

Surgical treatments for anal fissures aim to induce healing either by reducing anal tone (lateral sphincterotomy) or by direct advancement flap procedures with fissurectomy. If there is any concern regarding the aetiology of the fissure (eg. underlying malignancy or Crohn's' disease) or chronicity of the symptoms, then an EUA should be performed and biopsies taken.

Anal stretch is no longer used routinely due to the potential for significant sphincter damage and subsequent faecal incontinence. Botulinum toxin injection provides an adequate chemical sphincterotomy but is not currently first-line therapy.

Answer 16   A2, B1, C3, D4, E2

Dukes' staging is based on the histological examination of the resection specimen. A Dukes' A stage tumour is an invasive cancer that does not breach the muscularis propria. Dukes' B tumours breach the muscularis propria but regional lymph nodes are not involved. Dukes' C1 and C2 tumours involve lymph nodes, with the apical node negative and positive respectively. Dukes did not originally include a stage D. This additional clinical stage indicates the presence of distant metastases.

Answer 17   A3, B1, C4, D2, E5

Answer 18   A4, B1, C5, D3, E2

Peutz-Jegher's syndrome is an autosomal dominant inherited condition characterised by mucocutaneous pigmentation and multiple gastrointestinal hamartomatous polyps.

Over 80% of anal cancers are of squamous origin, arising from the squamous epithelium of the anal canal and perianal area. Colorectal cancers are almost exclusively adenocarcinomas that arise from the columnar epithelium.

Tubulovillous adenomas are pre-malignant lesions and once they exceed 1cm in diameter, the risk of malignancy rises to 5%. Larger adenomas are more likely to display cellular atypia (dysplasia) than smaller lesions.

Carcinoid tumours are found in between 1:100 and 1:1000 appendicectomy specimens. They are usually an incidental finding. The carcinoid syndrome is a very rare complication of appendiceal carcinoid.

Answer 19   A1, B1, C2, D1, E4

The lower vagina and labia drain into the superficial inguinal lymph nodes, as does the anus below the dentate line. Above the dentate line, the lymphatic vessels drain into the internal iliac lymph nodes.

The superficial inguinal nodes drain the skin of the buttock.

The sigmoid colon is drained by the inferior mesenteric lymph nodes.

Answer 20   A3, B5, C6, D4, (or 1 indirectly), E5, (or 1 indirectly)

Answer 21   A3, B4, C5, D2

Answer 22   A3, B1, C5, D4, E2

Answer 23   A5, B4, C2, D1, E5

Answer 24   A3, B2, C5, D3, E2

The foregut structures extend from the oesophagus to the site of the ampulla in the second part of the duodenum. The artery supplying this region is the coeliac artery.

The midgut includes the rest of the duodenum, all of the small bowel, and the colon up to the junction of the proximal two-thirds and distal third of the transverse colon. The superior mesenteric artery supplies the midgut structures.

The hindgut extends from the distal transverse colon to the rectum, and is supplied by the inferior mesenteric artery.

Answer 25   A6, B5, C2, D5, E1

After a total colectomy for colonic Crohn's disease, there is no colon remaining and the end of the small bowel is brought to the skin as a permanent spout ileostomy.

A patient who has undergone a low anterior resection with formation of a colon pouch after pre-operative radiotherapy is at a higher risk of anastomotic leakage than with other colorectal joins. Most surgeons would initially cover this type of anastomosis with a diversion loop ileostomy. The same is also true for restorative proctocolectomy.

Abdominoperineal resection involves resection of the distal colon and rectum, with removal of the anal canal. These patients have a permanent end colostomy.

In perforated diverticular disease, it is often considered unsafe to perform an anastomosis in the presence of significant sepsis. In these cases, a Hartmann's resection is carried out. The diseased segment of sigmoid colon is resected, the rectal stump is oversewn and a temporary colostomy fashioned. This stoma is potentially reversible at a later stage.

Answer 26   A3, B4, C1, D5, E2

Diverticular disease is a condition where acquired colonic diverticula are found, most commonly in the sigmoid colon. This is often an incidental finding and many patients with diverticular disease are asymptomatic.

Acute diverticulitis occurs when an infection arises in one or more diverticula. Patients often present with a few days' history of left iliac fossa pain associated with nausea and altered bowel habit. Acute phlegmonous diverticulitis is the result of a spreading low-grade cellulitis, mainly in the mesocolon. On abdominal examination the pelvic colon is tender and easily palpable, and the patient is usually unwell and pyrexial. If free perforation occurs from a ruptured diverticular abscess, the patient presents with signs of toxicity and general peritonitis. The most serious complication is faecal peritonitis.

A diverticular fistula arises when an inflamed diverticulum erodes into an adjacent viscus. The most common communications are colovesical and colovaginal, although fistulae have also been described between colon and appendix, fallopian tube, uterus, ureter and skin.

Answer 27   A1, B2, C6, D1, E3

The presence of colonic diverticula, especially in the sigmoid colon, is a common finding on barium enema and at colonoscopy. No action is required if this is an incidental finding and the patient is asymptomatic.

Resection of the diseased diverticular segment in an elective situation usually permits safe primary anastomosis of the colon. In the emergency situation where there is free perforation or faecal peritonitis, it is safer not to anastomose the bowel but to perform a Hartmann's resection after adequate resuscitation.

Percutaneous drainage of a pericolic abscess is an option for an unfit patient with localised signs.

Answer 28   A5, B5, C6, D1, E2

Answer 29   A5, B6, C1, D2

Answer 30   A4, B3, C5, D1, E2

Chapter 11

Urology

Damien Kelleher, FRCS
Staff Grade, Surgery, Morriston Hospital, Swansea, UK
Neil J Fenn, MB BCh FRCS (Ed) FRCS (Urol)
Consultant Urologist, Morriston Hospital, Swansea, UK

For all questions each option may be used once, more than once or not at all.

Question 1. Embryology

In to which structures do the following embryological ducts develop?

Options

1   Mesonephric (Wolffian) duct.
2   Paramesonephric (Mullerian) duct.

Stems

A   Develops into the uterus.
B   Forms the epididymus.
C   Incorporated into the developing bladder.
D   Persists as the prostatic utricle.
E   Remnants found in the broad ligament.

Question 2. Embryology

Match the dates with urinary tract developmental landmarks.

Options

1   18 days.
2   10 weeks.
3   18 weeks.
4   26 weeks.
5   36 weeks.

Stems

A   Testis decent begins.
B   First evidence of renal function.
C   Cloacal membrane develops at the caudal end of the 'primitive streak'.
D   Pelvic-ureteric junction identifiable.
E   Nephrogenesis complete.

Question 3. Anatomy

Regarding the abdominal wall.

Options

1   Transversalis fascia.
2   Campers fascia.
3   Scarpas fascia.
4   Conjoint tendon.
5   Rectus abdominis.

Stems

A   Covers the inner aspect of the transverse abdominis muscle.
B   Forms a distinct layer deep to Campers fascia.
C   Continuous with Colles fascia of the perineum.
D   Reinforces the posterior wall of the inguinal canal at the external ring.
E   Inserts on the xyphoid process and adjacent costal cartilages.

Question 4. Anatomy

Match the following statements to the corresponding vertebral level.

Options

1   T12.
2   L1.
3   L2.
4   L3.
5   L4.

Stems

A   Upper pole right kidney.
B   Upper pole left kidney.
C   Lower pole right kidney.
D   Lower pole left kidney.
E   Aortic bifurcation.

Question 5. Anatomy

Match the blood vessels with the correct statement.

Options

1   Aorta.
2   Gonadal artery.
3   Common iliac artery.
4   Pudendal artery.
5   Middle rectal artery.

Stems

A   Branches supply middle third of ureter.
B   Crosses anterior to ureter.
C   Passes posterior to ureter.
D   Is an area of anatomical ureteric narrowing.
E   Does not give any branches to the ureter.

Question 6. Anatomy

Concerning the branches of the internal iliac artery.

Options

1   Superior vesical artery.
2   Inferior vesical artery.
3   Obturator artery.
4   Internal pudendal artery.
5   Middle rectal artery.

Stems

A   Leaves pelvis through the greater sciatic foramen.
B   Distal end forms the medial umbilical ligament.
C   Passes lateral to the femoral ring.
D   Supplies the bladder trigone.
E   Terminal branches supply penis.

Question 7. Anatomy

Concerning pelvic nerves.

Options

1   Ilioinguinal nerve.
2   Obturator nerve.
3   Pelvic plexus nerves (parasympathetic fibres S2-4).
4   Hypogastric nerve (sympathetic fibres T11-L2).
5   Cavernosal nerves.

Stems

A   Responsible for ejaculation.
B   Stimulate detrusor contraction.
C   Damage results in weak hip adduction.
D   Supplies skin of scrotum or labia majora.
E   Required for penile tumescence.

Question 8. Anatomy

Which structure drains primarily to the following lymph node groups?

Options

1   Para-aortic/lumbar lymph nodes.
2   Superficial inguinal lymph nodes.
3   External iliac lymph nodes.
4   Cloquet's node.
5   Obturator nodes.

Stems

A   Testis.
B   Epididymus.
C   Prostate gland.
D   Anterior abdominal wall.
E   Penile skin.

Question 9. Physiology

Regarding renal physiology.

Options

1   Proximal convoluted tubule (PCT).
2   Glomerulus.
3   Distal convoluted tubule (DCT).
4   Loop of Henle.
5   Collecting duct.

Stems

A   Determines final urinary sodium concentration.
B   Thiazide diuretics exert their effect at this section of the nephron.
C   Has the greatest concentration gradient.
D   Is antidiuretic hormone (ADH) sensitive.
E   Is responsible for the majority of sodium reabsorbtion.

Question 10. Physiology

Match each compound with the correct statement.

Options

1   Renin.
2   Angiotensin I.
3   Angiotensin II.
4   Angiotensinogen.
5   Aldosterone.

Stems

A   Production leads directly to sodium loss.
B   Is secreted by the juxta-glomerular apparatus.
C   Is a protease.
D   Is only produced in the kidney.
E   Is pharmacologically inactive.

Question 11. Physiology

Correctly match the following substances with the correct statement.

Options

1   Luteinising hormone (LH).
2   Follicle stimulating hormone (FSH).
3   Dihydrotestosterone (DHT).
4   Testosterone.
5   Oestrogen.

Stems

A   Is secreted by Leydig cells.
B   Acts upon Leydig cells.
C   Regulates testosterone production.
D   Is produced by the action of 5α reductase.
E   Initiates spermatogenesis.

Question 12. Physiology

Match the following statements with the appropriate incidence.

Options

1   0.9%.
2   2.6%.
3   60%.
4   85%.
5   98%.

Stems

A   Incidence of foetal urinary tract abnormalities.
B   Prevalence of genitourinary tuberculosis in the United Kingdom.
C   Bound testosterone in plasma.
D   Renal stones containing calcium oxalate.
E   Prostate carcinoma originating from the peripheral zone.

Question 13. Microbiology

Match the statements regarding common urinary bacteria.

Options

1   Mycobacterium tuberculosis.
2   Escherichia Coli.
3   Bacteroides fragilis.
4   Pseudomonas aerugenosa.
5   Proteus mirabilis.

Stems

A   Is an obligate anaerobe.
B   Causes the urine to become alkaline.
C   Commonest community urinary tract infection pathogen.
D   Commonly associated with staghorn calculus formation.
E   Is an acid fast bacillus.

on 14. Microbiology

ɘrning urinary tract infections (UTIs).

Options

1   A uromucoid modulating bacterial attachment.
2   Bacterial filamentous protein appendages.
3   Bagged or clean catch specimen.
4   Midstream urine collection.
5   Dipstick urine test for white blood cells in the urine.

Stems

A   Mannose sensitive (type 1) pili.
B   Leucocyte esterase.
C   Tamm-Horsfall protein.
D   Standard urine collection method in adults.
E   Used in the neonate.

Question 15. Pharmacology

Mode of action of common antibiotics used for infections in the urinary tract.

Options

1   Trimethoprim.
2   Nitrofurantoin.
3   Ciprofloxacin.
4   Gentamycin.
5   Amoxicillin.

Stems

A   Inhibits DNA gyrase.
B   Inhibits protein wall synthesis.
C   Antagonises folate synthesis.
D   Is ototoxic.
E   Inhibits ribosomal RNA synthesis.

Question 16. Pharmacology

Match the drug class with the appropriate response.

Options

1   α-agonist.
2   α-antagonist.
3   5 α-reductase inhibitor.
4   β-antagonist.
5   Anti-cholinergic.

Stems

A   Reduction of bladder outflow obstruction.
B   Retrograde ejaculation.
C   Detumesence of priapism.
D   Reduction in prostatic size.
E   Reduces unstable bladder contractions.

Question 17. Imaging

Match the investigations with the statement.

Options

1   Positron emission tomography (PET).
2   Ultrasound scan (USS).
3   Computed tomography (CT).
4   Intravenous pyelogram (IVP).
5   Magnetic resonance imaging (MRI).

Stems

A   Scanning based on the uptake of fluorodeoxyglucose.
B   Generates images by transducer emitted short burst of pulsed sound waves.
C   Utilises alignment of hydrogen protons forming magnetic vectors.
D   Requires simultaneous tube rotation and continuous x-ray exposure.
E   Uses tomogram to help delineate abnormalities.

Question 18. Imaging

Match the contrast agents/radionucleotides to the appropriate investigation.

Options

1   Technetium 99 Mercaptoacetyl triglycine (MAG3).
2   Technetium 99 Dimercaptosuccinic acid (DMSA).
3   Technetium 99 Methyldiphosphonate (MDP).
4   Low osmolality contrast media (eg. Iohexol or Iopamidol).
5   Gadolinium-DTPA.

Stems

A   Agent of choice for renal cortical imaging.
B   Agent used for intravenous pyelogram.
C   Predominantly cleared by tubular secretion.
D   Paramagnetic contrast agent.
E   Imaging skeletal metastases.

Question 19. Haematuria

For each of the following patients with haematuria, select the MOST likely diagnosis.

Options

1   Bladder transitional cell cancer.
2   Bladder stones.
3   Interstitial cystitis.
4   Glomerulonephritis.
5   Traumatic perinephric haematoma.
6   Prostate cancer.
7   Renal cell cancer.
8   Secondary haemorrhage.
9   Staghorn calculus.
10   Ureteric transition cell cancer.
11   Urinary tract infection.

Stems

A An 18-year-old sexually active female presents with intermittent episodes of frequency, urgency, dysuria and microscopic haematuria. Some episodes are associated with suprapubic and bilateral loin pain. Clinical examination and renal tract imaging were normal.

B A 55-year-old male presented with weight loss, anorexia, night sweats and macroscopic haematuria. He was noted to have a raised ESR and polycythaemia.

C A 78-year-old male presents with macroscopic haematuria and clot retention. Ten days prior to this he had undergone a transurethral resection of the prostate for long-standing lower urinary tract symptoms.

D A 26-year-old female became generally unwell 3 weeks after a sore throat. She was noted to be hypertensive. Urine analysis showed microscopic haematuria and proteinuria.

E A 60-year-old male presents with an episode of painless macroscopic haematuria. Clinical examination was normal. He is a life-long smoker of 20 cigarettes a day.

Question 20. Scrotal swelling

Match the statements with the most likely scrotal swelling diagnosis.

Options

1 Varicocoele.
2 Hydrocoele.
3 Sperm granuloma.
4 Inguinal hernia.
5 Testicular malignancy.

Stems

A   A 65-year-old man with a soft transilluminable swelling confined to the scrotum.

B   A 25-year-old man with a painless, firm testicular swelling.

C   A 36-year-old man with a painful nodule within the spermatic cord following a vasectomy.

D   A 32-year-old man with a soft mass around the left testicle which is more pronounced on standing.

E   A 52-year-old man with a smooth painless symmetrical right inguinal-scrotal swelling. Positive cough impulse.

Question 21. Sexually transmitted diseases

Options

1   *Neisseria gonorrhoeae.*
2   *Chlamydia trachomatis.*
3   Herpes simplex virus.
4   Syphilis.
5   Scabies.

Stems

A   Infective agent in Lymphogranuloma venereum.

B   Presents with a painless genital sore 2-4 weeks after exposure.

C   Common cause of epididymitis in heterosexual men under 35 years of age.

D   Treated with permethrin cream.

E   Diagnosis via culture of wound fluid or serum antigen testing.

Question 22. Appropriate antibiotic use

Match the most appropriate antibiotic for use as first-line treatment for the following clinical settings.

Options

1   Ofloxacin.
2   Trimethoprim.
3   Doxycycline.
4   Penicillin V.
5   Gentamycin.

Stems

A   A 49-year-old man diagnosed with acute prostatitis.
B   A 21-year-old girl diagnosed with genitourinary Chlamydia.
C   A 25-year-old man who had a splenectomy for traumatic rupture 12 months before.
D   A 34-year-old woman with a 1-day history of dysuria and urinary frequency.
E   A 30-year-old man diagnosed with gonorrhoea.

Question 23. Priapism

Match the clinical setting with the most likely type of priapism.

Options

1   High flow.
2   Low flow.

Stems

A   Corporal ischaemia and damage may occur after just 6 hours of priapism.
B   A 20-year-old African man with sickle cell anaemia and a 4-hour history of priapism.
C   An 18-year-old man with a penetrating injury to the perineum and priapism.
D   Painless priapism.
E   Treatment may require embolisation or ligation.

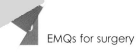

Question 24. Consent issues

Which of the following statements concerning full informed consent are true?

Options

1　A young person of any age can give a valid consent to treatment or examination provided that he/she is considered competent to make the decision.

2　Separate consent is required for research procedures.

3　All adults aged 16 and over are presumed, in law, to have capacity to consent to treatment unless there is evidence to the contrary.

4　Patient consent is required on every occasion a doctor wishes to initiate an examination, treatment or other intervention, except in emergencies or where the law prescribes.

5　The BMA considers the doctor who recommends that the patient should undergo the intervention should have responsibility for providing an explanation to the patient and obtaining his/her consent.

Stems

A　1 and 2.
B　1, 3 and 5.
C　3, 4 and 5.
D　1, 2, 3 and 4.
E　1, 2, 3, 4 and 5.

Question 25. Procedure

Link the following procedures to the recognised complication.

Options

1　Vasectomy.
2　Transurethral resection of the prostate (TURP).
3　Transurethral resection of bladder tumour (TURBT).
4　Radical nephrectomy.
5　Radical prostatectomy.

Stems

A   TUR syndrome.
B   Splenic laceration.
C   Impotence.
D   Sperm granuloma.
E   Obturator nerve stimulation (obturator kick).

Question 26. Urinary tract symptoms

When calculating AUA/IPSS scores for patients with lower urinary tract symptoms, which statements are true or false?

Options

1   True.
2   False.

Stems

A   Involves administration of questionnaire by medically trained person.
B   Consists of 7 questions each scoring up to 5 points.
C   Are disease-specific.
D   Pivotal in research into new treatments.
E   Clear trend between increasing age and symptom score.

Question 27. Urinary tract symptoms

For each of the following patients with lower urinary tract symptoms, select the MOST likely diagnosis.

Options

1   Acontractile bladder.
2   Benign prostatic hypertrophy.
3   Bladder neck stenosis.
4   Hyper-reflexia with detrusor striated sphincter dyssynergia (DSSD).
5   Diabetes mellitus.
6   Genuine stress incontinence.
7   Low pressure-low flow voiding.
8   Multiple sclerosis.
9   Parkinsons disease.
10 Spinal canal stenosis.
11 Urethral stricture.

Stems

A   A 70-year-old male presents with a 5-year history of a poor flow, hesitancy, frequency, nocturia and post-micturition dribbling. A flow rate showed a Qmax of 7mls/sec with a voided volume of 270mls and a residual of 100mls.

B   A 40-year-old female presents with urinary incontinence when coughing, sneezing and during her fitness class. She has had 3 children delivered vaginally. The first labour was prolonged and required repair of a second degree tear.

C   A 16-year-old male presents with a long history of hesitancy and worsening urinary stream. He also complains of post-micturition dribbling, which may occur some minutes after he completes his normal void. He had a significant fall astride injury as a child.

D   A 40-year-old women presents with urinary frequency, urgency and episodes of urge incontinence. She had a transient episode of unilateral blindness 2 years prior to these new symptoms.

E   A 20-year-old male suffered a supra-sacral spinal cord injury in a RTA. He was initially managed with an indwelling catheter and then commenced on intermittent self-catheterisation. In between episodes of catheterisation he complains of urinary incontinence.

Question 28. Urodynamics

Match the following urodynamics traces with the diagnosis.

Options

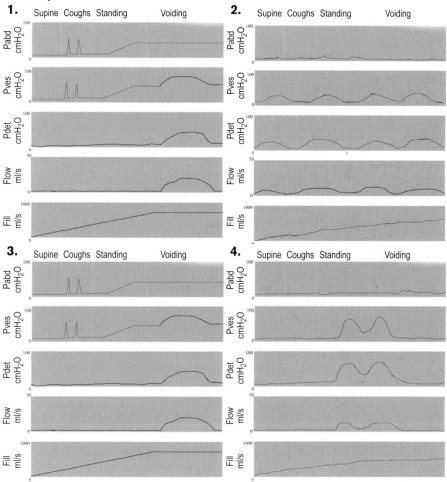

Stems

A Detrusor instability.
B Stress incontinence.
C Normal.
D Hyper-reflexia.

Question 29. Urinary diversion

Options

1   Ileal conduit.
2   Mitrofanoff principle.
3   Nephrostomy tube.
4   Ureterosigmoidostomy.
5   Clam enterocystoplasty.

Stems

A   Hypokalemia is more common than in any other type of urinary diversion.
B   Temporary urinary diversion.
C   Utilises catheterisable stoma.
D   Parastomal hernia is a well-recognised problem.
E   Uses 10-15cm of terminal ileum.

Question 30. Renal stones

Match the stone composition with the most likely clinical findings.

Options

1   Calcium oxalate.
2   Calcium phosphate.
3   Uric acid.
4   Ammonium magnesium phosphate.
5   Cysteine stones.

Stems

A   Radiolucent stone on plain x-ray.
B   Associated with *Proteus mirabalis* infections.
C   Associated with renal tubular acidosis.
D   Associated with inherited defective brush border transport mechanism.
E   Most common stone composition in the UK.

Question 31. Renal stones

In the treatment of renal stones.

Options

1 No active treatment.
2 Lithotripsy (ESWL).
3 Ureteroscopic extraction with fragmentation.
4 Percutaneous nephrolithotomy.
5 Open nephrolithotomy.

Stems

A 1cm stone in lower pole calyx.
B Partial staghorn calculus.
C 3mm stone at vesico-ureteric junction.
D 1cm lower ureteric stone.
E Renal stone with associated PUJ obstruction.

Question 32. Ureteric obstruction

In the following causes of ureteric obstruction, correctly pair the following.

Options

1 Radiotherapy.
2 Retroperitoneal fibrosis.
3 Ureteric calculus.
4 Iatrogenic.
5 Ureteric transitional cell tumour.

Stems

A Ureters are often medially displaced.
B Obstruction is bilateral in 15% (and most common after pelvic surgery).
C 30% of patients will have a non-functioning kidney at presentation.
D Is caused by a reduction in the ureteric vascular supply.
E May respond to steroid therapy.

Question 33. Undescended testes

Options

1   True.
2   False.

Stems

A   Incidence at birth is 3%.
B   Bilateral in 15% of cases.
C   Should not be treated until the age of 5.
D   Associated with an increased risk of testicular cancer.
E   No associated increased risk of torsion.

Question 34. Urological tumour markers

Options

1   Prostatic specific antigen (PSA).
2   Lactate dehydrogenase (LDH).
3   Alpha feto protein (α-FP).
4   Beta human chorionic gonadotrophin (β-HCG).
5   Placental alkaline phosphatase (PLAP).

Stems

A   Has age-specific ranges.
B   Produced by syncytiotrophoblast cells in germ cell tumours.
C   A ubiquitous cellular enzyme which is useful for monitoring germ cell tumours.
D   A 32 kiloDalton serine protease.
E   Associated with carcinoma of the testes, liver and pancreas.

Question 35. Renal lesions

Match up the following statements relating to renal lesions.

Options

1   Clear cell cancers.
2   Von Hippel-Lindau disease.
3   Oncocytoma.
4   Angiomyolipoma.
5   Familial papillary renal cancer.

Stems

A   50% of patients with tuberous sclerosis have these lesions.
B   Commonest renal cancer cell type.
C   Rare familial syndrome with tumours of the kidney, cerebellum and retina.
D   Contains fat, muscle and vascular components.
E   Difficult to differentiate from renal cell cancer.

Question 36. Prostate cancer treatment

Options

1   Radiotherapy.
2   Active surveillance.
3   Brachytherapy.
4   Radical prostatectomy.
5   Hormone manipulation.

Stems

A   Involves the implantation of radioactive seeds.
B   May be used to treat asymptomatic elderly patients.
C   Can be used to treat localised disease and symptomatic metastasis.
D   May produce hot flushes.
E   Bilateral nerve-sparing is performed with this treatment.

Question 37. Staging

Local staging of prostate cancer.

Options

1   T1a
2   T1b
3   T1c
4   T2a
5   T2b
6   T3a
7   T3b
8   T4

Stems

A   A 56-year-old man who requests a PSA test from his GP. This comes back at 7ng/ml. He has a normal DRE, but a needle biopsy confirms prostate cancer.

B   A 50-year-old man underwent a radical prostatectomy. On histological examination, the prostate cancer involved the right lobe as well as the right seminal vesical.

C   An 85-year-old man who had a TURP for bladder outflow symptoms. The histology showed prostatic adenocarcinoma involving 3% of 'chippings'.

D   A 72-year-old man was seen in the OPD with mild bladder outflow symptoms. His PSA is 8ng/ml and he has a hard nodule in the left lobe of his prostate.

E   A 90-year-old man was admitted with retention of urine. His PSA was 263ng/ml. DRE revealed a large prostate tumour fixed to the pelvis side wall.

Question 38. Treatment

Match the following compounds with the appropriate statement.

Options

1 Finasteride.
2 LHRH analogues.
3 Diethylstilboestrol.
4 Testosterone.
5 Flutamide.

Stems

A Marked thromboembolic effect.
B Is used in the treatment of BPH.
C Blocks the androgen receptor.
D May cause 'flare' phenomenon.
E Not used to treat prostate cancer.

Question 39. Treatment of testicular cancer

Options

1 Seminoma - Stage I.
2 Seminoma - Stage IIa.
3 Seminoma - Stage III.
4 Teratoma - Stage I.
5 Teratoma - Stage III.

Stems

A 5-year survival rates of 95%.
B Orchidectomy platinum-based chemotherapy.
C Ochidectomy and adjuvant radiotherapy.
D Orchidectomy and surveillance only.
E Bleomycin, etoposide and cisplatin-based chemotherapy.

Question 40. Bladder cancer

Bladder cancer in the UK.

Options

1 Number of patients with squamous cell cancer on histology.
2 Number of patients with superficial disease who subsequently progress.
3 Number of patients with invasive disease at presentation.
4 Number of patients with superficial disease at presentation.
5 Number of patients with transitional cell cancer on histology.

Stems

A 1%.
B 10%.
C 20%.
D 80%.
E 90%.

Answer 1   A2, B1, C1, D2, E1

The mesonephric duct in the male is linked to the testes by persistent mesonephric tubules. The lower end is taken in by the bladder to become part of the trigone. The remainder forms the epididymus, vas deferens, seminal vesicles and ejaculatory ducts. In the female, remnants of the mesonephric duct may be found in the broad ligament. The paramesonephric duct develops immediately lateral to the mesonephric duct. It is important in the female forming the fallopian tubes and fusing in the midline to form the uterine body and cervix. Failure or incomplete fusion will produce congenital abnormalities of the uterus.

Answer 2   A4, B2, C1, D3, E5

Answer 3   A1, B3, C3, D4, E5

Answer 4   A2, B1, C4, D4, E5

Answer 5   A2, B2, C3, D3, E4

Answer 6   A4, B1, C3, D2, E4

The renal and gonadal arteries are paired arteries arising from the aorta. The ureter receives segmental supply from various sources (renal artery, gonadal artery, aorta, common iliac and branches of the internal iliac artery). The remainder of the pelvic organs are supplied by the internal iliac vessels.

The common iliac artery bifurcates into the external and internal iliac arteries at the sacro-iliac joints. The internal iliac artery descends into the pelvis and divides into anterior and posterior trunks. The anterior trunk gives off seven (superior vesical, middle rectal, inferior vesicle, uterine artery, internal pudendal, obturator and inferior gluteal artery) branches whilst the posterior trunk gives off three (superior gluteal, ascending lumbar and lateral sacral) branches.

Answer 7   A4, B3, C2, D1, E5

Answer 8   A1, B1, C5, D3, E2

The penis, scrotum and perineum drain into the inguinal nodes, which communicate through the femoral ring and Cloquet's node to external iliac nodes. The testes and epididymus drain directly to the para-aortic nodes.

In the pelvis there are 3 major groups of lymph nodes associated with the major vessels (common, internal and external iliac). The majority of the pelvis viscera drain through the internal iliac nodes and their tributaries (presacral, obturator and internal pudendal nodes). The common iliac nodes receive efferents from both internal and external chains prior to draining into the lateral aortic nodes.

Answer 9   A5, B3, C4, D5, E1

Blood is filtered at the glomerulus. The PCT is responsible for reabsorption of 95% of electrolytes. The DCT is responsible for the 'fine tuning' of electrolytes where thiazide diuretics exert their effect. The loop of Henle descends into the high osmolality medulla which allows reabsorption of water along its concentration gradient. ADH increases water permeability in the ascending part.

Answer 10   A5, B1, C1, D1, E2

When arterial blood pressure or blood volume decreases, perfusion of the juxtaglomerular apparatus in the kidneys is reduced. In response the juxtaglomerular cells of the afferent arteriole release the enzyme renin. Renin cleaves the inactive peptide called angiotensinogen, converting it into angiotensin I. Angiotensin I is converted to angiotensin II by the angiotensin converting enzyme (ACE), which is found mainly in lung capillaries. Although angiotensin I may have some minor activity, angiotensin II is a more powerful vasoconstrictor and facilitates the release of aldosterone. Longer-term actions include vascular growth and ventricular hypertrophy.

Answer 11   A4, B1, C1, D3, E2

In the testes, LH binds to receptors on Leydig cells, stimulating synthesis and secretion of testosterone. The steroid sex hormone testosterone is converted to its more active form dihydrotestosterone by the enzyme 5α reductase.

FSH is required for normal sperm production. It supports the function of Sertoli cells, which in turn support many aspects of sperm cell maturation.

Answer 12   A1, B2, C5, D3, E4

Answer 13   A3, B5, C2, D5, E1

Most urinary tract infections are caused by facultative anaerobes that are able to grow either under anaerobic or aerobic conditions and originate in the bowel flora. *E.coli* is the commonest urinary pathogen accounting for 85% of community-acquired and 50% of hospital-acquired infections. Fastidious organisms such as *Bacteroides fragilis* (an obligate anaerobe) and Chlamydia can also cause infections of the urinary tract. Mycobacteria species do not stain with the Gram stain and composition of their cell wall makes them 'acid fast'.

Answer 14   A2, B5, C1, D4, E5

Answer 15   A3, B5, C1, D4, E4

DNA gyrase is an essential bacterial enzyme that catalyzes super-coiling of double-stranded closed-circular DNA. The key event in quinolone action is reversible trapping of the gyrase-DNA complex. Trimethoprim is a bactericidal antibiotic which acts by interfering with the action of bacterial dihydrofolate reductase, inhibiting synthesis of tetrahydrofolic acid. Aminoglycosides' mode of action is via inhibition of ribosomal protein synthesis. Ototoxicity is a well recognised side effect of gentamicin. The mechanism of aminoglycoside ototoxicity remains unknown, but it appears to involve both apoptotic pathways as well as formation of free radicals.

Answer 16   A2, B2, C1, D3, E5

Alpha-1-adrenergic receptor blockers inhibit contraction of prostatic and bladder neck smooth muscle. Phenylephrine, an alpha-agonist, is useful in the management of iatrogenic priapism via sympathomimetic vasopressor activity.

5α reductase converts testosterone to the more active dihydrotestosterone (DHT). DHT is the primary mediator of prostate growth.

Anticholinergic compounds cause relaxation of bladder smooth muscle and have an effect on the overactive bladder.

Answer 17   A1, B2, C5, D3, E4

Answer 18   A2, B4, C1, D4, E3

Dimercaptosuccinic acid (DMSA) is taken up and bound firmly by the renal cortex. Mercaptoacetyl triglycine (MAG3) is cleared primarily by tubular secretion and thus estimates renal plasma flow, and which itself corresponds to differential renal function. In the case of MDP, the radiopharmaceutical becomes concentrated in areas of bone turnover (eg. a fracture, neoplasm and osteoarthritis). Gadolinium polarizes the binding between hydrogen and oxygen. This causes an enhanced magnetic moment which outlines tissues during MRI scans.

Answer 19   A11, B7, C8, D4, E1

Answer 20   A2, B5, C3, D1, E4

Haematuria (both micro- and macroscopic), scrotal swellings and raised serum prostatic specific antigen (PSA) are all considered important indicators of possible underlying malignancy and are thus covered by the '10-day rule'. Guidelines, produced by the local 'cancer network' should be available to standardise the investigation of these symptoms.

Answer 21   A2, B4, C2, D5, E3

Answer 22   A1, B3, C4, D2, E1

The organisms most commonly involved in prostatitis are: *Escherichia coli*, *Streptococcus faecalis* and *Staphylococcus aureus* which are all sensitive to ofloxacin. The quinolones have good prostatic penetrance. Tetracyclines are the antibiotic of choice for *Chlamydia trachomatis*. Traditionally, doxycycline was used as it can be taken with food, and is inexpensive. Due to a compliance issue single-dose preparations are now available. Post-splenectomy cover against *Streptococcus pneumoniae*, *Haemophilus influenzae* and *Neisseria meningitides* is recommended for the first 2 years. For uncomplicated UTI trimethoprim 200mg BD for 3 days is recommended.

Answer 23   A2, B2, C1, D1, E1

In high-flow priapism there is an arterial-venous fistula leading to a continuous high flow of oxygen-rich blood through the penis, so it is painless and does not cause long-term damage. In low-flow priapism the drainage of blood from the penis is impaired leaving the shaft of the penis filled with deoxygenated venous blood with potential for hypoxic damage.

Answer 24   E

A tool kit for consent is available from the BMA on www.bma.org.uk.

Answer 25   A2, B4, C4, D1, E3

Answer 26   A2, B1, C2, D1, E1

Answer 27   A2, B6, C11, D8, E4

Answer 28   A2, B4, C1, D3

Answer 29   A4, B3, C2, D1, E1

Answer 30   A3, B4, C2, D5, E1

Answer 31   A2, B4, C1, D3, E5

The treatment of upper tract stones has undergone dramatic changes since the 1980s due to the development of lithotripsy, percutaneous access and ureteroscopic equipment advances. Open surgery now has a limited role. Treatment options will also depend on stone size, composition, location, renal anatomy and local availability.

Answer 32   A2, B4, C2, D1, E2

Answer 33   A1, B1, C2, D1, E2

Answer 34   A1, B4, C2, D1, E3

Answer 35   A4, B1, C2, D4, E3

Answer 36   A3, B2, C1, D5, E4

Answer 37   A3, B7, C1, D4, E8

Classification of malignant disease allows treatment planning and prognosis estimation. The TNM Classification is the most widely used system for classiying the extent of cancer spread. The most up-to-date classification can be found in *AJCC cancer staging manual*. Lippincott, Philadelphia, 1977.

Answer 38   A3, B1, C5, D2, E4

Diethylstilboestrol is a useful adjunct in advanced prostatic cancer, but causes enhancement of blood coagulation by increased circulating factors II, VII, IX, X, decreased antithrombin III, increased plasminogen concentration and decreased platelet adhesiveness. Finasteride inhibits 5α reductase (which converts testosterone into its more active form) and thus, causes a decrease in prostatic volume. Flutamide is a non-steroidal anti-androgen. Initial administration of LHRH analogues can cause a surge in tumour growth before suppression occurs.

Answer 39   A1, B3, C1, D4, E5

Answer 40   A1, B2, C3, D4, E5

Chapter 12
Orthopaedics & trauma

Paul Williams, BSc (Hons) MB BCh FRCS (Eng) FRCS Tr & Orth
Consultant Trauma & Orthopaedic Surgeon
Stuart Roy, MB ChB MPhil (Cantab) FRCS (Ed) Tr & Orth
Specialist Registrar, Trauma & Orthopaedics
Morriston Hospital, Swansea, UK

For all questions each option may be used once, more than once or not at all.

Question 1. Fractures of the distal radius

Match the most suitable management strategy for the following patients.

Options

1   Displaced, comminuted Colles' fracture.
2   Unstable Smith's fracture.
3   Taurus fracture.
4   Displaced Salter Harris 2 fracture.
5   Galleazi fracture in an adult.

Stems

A   Application of POP and review in clinic in 3 weeks.
B   Manipulation +/- k-wiring in theatre.
C   Treat fracture appropriately and screen for osteoporosis.
D   Volar buttress plate application.
E   Plating of radius and screening of distal radio-ulna joint (DRUJ).

Question 2. Fractured neck of femur

For each fracture choose the single most appropriate operation.

Options

1 Take to theatre within 6 hours to reduce and fix the fracture.
2 Cannulated screw fixation.
3 Take to theatre to reduce fracture and hold reduction with a dynamic hip screw (DHS).
4 Bipolar hemiarthroplasty.
5 Cementless hemiarthroplasty.

Stems

A Minimally displaced sub-capital fracture in an 82-year-old lady.
B Completely displaced sub-capital fracture in a 94-year-old lady with significant medical co-morbidity who is minimally mobile.
C Completely displaced sub-capital fracture in a fit 65-year-old man.
D Three part inter-trochanteric fracture in a 72-year-old male.
E Displaced sub-capital fracture in a 45-year-old male.

Question 3. Acute knee injuries

Match the most appropriate management option to the clinical scenario.

Options

1 Reduction of joint and emergency angiography.
2 Rest knee in pop cylinder for 6 weeks and then physiotherapy.
3 X-ray, aspirate joint, if no fracture seen brace for 6 weeks, physiotherapy and refer for MRI scan.
4 Admit, x-ray +/- ultrasound scan, theatre for direct repair patellar tendon with wire loop protection.
5 Admit, x-ray, EUA and arthroscopy.

Stems

A   First time dislocation of the patella playing football, relocated on the pitch.

B   Dislocated knee with pale, cold foot following rugby tackle.

C   Twisted knee playing rugby with swelling within 2 hours of injury.

D   Injured knee playing football, unable to straighten the knee, fixed flexion of 30 degrees.

E   55-year-old man mowing lawn on a slope, felt 'something go' and now unable to straighten leg.

Question 4. Management of back pain

For each of the following causes of back pain choose the most appropriate option.

Options

1   Oblique x-rays, CT scan +/- bone scan.

2   X-ray, dietary advice and lifestyle advice and physiotherapy.

3   Urgent investigation including x-ray, MRI, and bloods with electrophoresis.

4   Urgent investigation and theatre.

5   Urgent investigation with bloods and a bone scan.

Stems

A   Low back pain in a 15-year-old gymnast.

B   Low back pain associated with night sweats and weight loss.

C   Chronic low back pain with sudden increase associated with incontinence of urine and saddle anaesthesia.

D   Chronic low back pain in an obese, middle-aged lady who smokes.

E   Mid-thoracic pain in a 10-year-old girl.

Question 5. Septic arthritis

Match the appropriate option(s) to the stems below.

Options

1 Aspirate and send for microbiology and sensitivity.
2 Aspirate the joint in theatre and proceed to formal open washout if indicated.
3 Surgical washout followed by 1 week of IV antibiotics followed by 6 weeks of oral antibiotics.
4 Serial ESR and CRP measurements are useful markers of improvement.
5 Repeat visits to theatre may be necessary.

Stems

A Gradual swelling of knee post-arthroscopy with associated pain and pyrexia.
B Systemically unwell infant with severe pain in left hip.
C 65-year-old lady on ITU with chest infection presents with hot, swollen right knee.
D 75-year-old lady on steroids presents with hot, swollen wrist.
E 23-year-old male punched someone in the mouth 2 days previously and presents with a 'mucky' looking laceration over his right 4th metacarpophalangeal joint (MCPJ).

Question 6. Open fractures

Choose the most appropriate Gustilo & Anderson grading for the following clinical scenarios.

Options

1 Motorcyclist at 60mph hitting wall and sustaining open distal tibial fracture with a 2-3cm inside-out wound and no bone exposed.
2 Footballer tackling goalkeeper sustaining open distal tibial fracture with 5cm wound, bone exposed and periosteal stripping.
3 72-year-old lady falling on outstretched hand with Colles' fracture and puncture wound <1cm over ulnar styloid.

4   Driver cut from car involved in head-on RTA with 5cm wound over distal tibial fracture and pulseless foot.

5   Driver cut from the other car involved in the RTA with 10cm wound over femoral fracture, no bone exposed, adequate soft tissue coverage and no periosteal stripping.

6   Student falling off kerb sustaining 2-3cm wound over open ankle fracture with moderate soft-tissue damage.

Stems

A   Grade I.
B   Grade II.
C   Grade IIIa.
D   Grade IVb.
E   Grade Vc.

Question 7. Compartment syndrome

Choose the most suitable management strategy for the following patients.

Options

1   Ventilated multiple trauma patient following intramedullary nailing of tibia.

2   Off-ended proximal radius and ulnar fracture following manipulation under anaesthesia (MUA) in a 4-year-old boy.

3   Chronic exertional lower limb pain.

4   Circumferential full thickness neck burns.

5   Closed distal tibial fracture with passive stretch pain to extension hallux.

6   Open distal tibial fracture with passive stretch pain to hallux.

Stems

A   Emergency fasciotomy.
B   Elective fasciotomy.
C   Emergency escharotomy.
D   Regular clinical neurovascular observational review.
E   Formal compartment pressure monitoring.

Question 8. Fracture names

Choose the area of the body in which the following named fractures occur.

Options

1 Tear drop fracture.
2 Lisfranc fracture dislocation.
3 Jones fracture.
4 Monteggia fracture.
5 Chance fracture.
6 Malgaigne fractures.

Stems

A Upper limb.
B Lower limb.
C Pelvis.
D Spine.

Question 9. Fracture classification

Choose the most suitable classification system to aid description of the clinical scenario.

Options

1 Displaced distal radial epiphyseal injury in a 6-year-old boy.
2 Displaced intracapsular fracture neck of femur in a 78-year-old lady.
3 Displaced lateral malleolar fracture in a 22-year-old professional footballer.
4 Displaced acetabular fracture.
5 Depressed lateral tibial plateau fracture.

Stems

A Weber classification.
B Schatzker classification.
C Salter Harris classification.
D Garden classification.
E Letournel classification.

Question 10. Total hip replacement

Choose the most appropriate statement for the following options.

Options

1 The nerve most at risk is the lateral cutaneous nerve of thigh.
2 Supplies the majority of blood to the femoral head.
3 Preserves the gluteus medius leading to a decrease in postoperative lurch.
4 The superior gluteal nerve is at risk with this approach.
5 Confers more stability for a total hip replacement.

Stems

A The posterior approach to the hip.
B Placement of the femoral prosthesis in retroversion.
C The anterior approach to the hip.
D Medial circumflex femoral artery.
E Hardinge approach to the hip.

Question 11. Total knee replacement

The following statements relate to which particular aspect of total knee replacement?

Options

1 Very stable joint replacement.
2 The peroneal nerve is at risk.
3 Requires the presence of the anterior cruciate ligament.
4 There is a higher risk of infection.
5 The results are excellent at 10-year follow-up.

Stems

A A hinged total knee replacement.
B Unicompartmental knee replacement.
C Replacing the valgus knee.
D Knee replacement for psoriatic arthropathy.
E Rotating platform knee replacement.

Question 12. Nerve entrapment / brachial plexus

Match the nerve/nerve roots with the following.

Options

1   Common peroneal nerve.
2   C5, 6.
3   C7, 8, T1.
4   Median nerve.
5   Radial nerve.

Stems

A   Saturday night palsy.
B   Carpal tunnel syndrome.
C   Foot drop.
D   Erb's palsy.
E   Klumpke's palsy.

Question 13. Arthritis

Choose the relevant radiological feature/s to match the following conditions.

Options

1   Joint space narrowing.
2   Periarticular erosions.
3   Pencil-in-cup deformity.
4   Non-marginal syndesmophytes.
5   Gross disorganisation of the affected joint.

Stems

A   Psoriatic arthropathy.
B   Charcot arthropathy.
C   Osteoarthritis.
D   Rheumatoid arthritis.
E   Ankylosing spondylitis.

Question 14. Hallux valgus

Choose the most suitable management option for the following patients.

Options

1   30-year-old female with painful bunion, normal 1st metatarsophalangeal joint (MTPJ) and hallux valgus (HV) angle.
2   75-year-old man with very painful, degenerate 1st MTPJ.
3   48-year-old lady with HV angle of 30 degrees and intermetatrsal angle of 18 degrees.
4   40-year-old lady with HV angle of 24 degrees and normal intermetatarsal angle.
5   78-year-old lady with painful hallux valgus; lives in a residential home.

Stems

A   Trial of shoe change followed by a Keller's hemiarthroplasty.
B   Trial of shoe change followed by exostectomy.
C   Distal 1st metatarsal osteotomy.
D   Proximal 1st metatarsal osteotomy +/- distal soft tissue procedure.
E   Fusion of 1st MTPJ.

Question 15. Paediatrics

Choose the physical findings that can be exhibited in the following childhood conditions.

Options

1   Limp.
2   Knee pain.
3   Leg length discrepancy.
4   Torn frenulum.
5   Obligatory external rotation in flexion.

Stems

A   Perthes' disease.
B   Slipped Capital Femoral Epiphysis (SCFE).
C   Developmental dysplasia of the hip (DDH).
D   Osgood Schlatter's disease.
E   Non-accidental injury.

Question 16. Metabolic bone disease

For each of the following abnormalities select the appropriate disorder/s.

Options

1   Looser's zones on radiographs.
2   Metaphyseal cupping on radiographs.
3   Pathological fracture.
4   Long bone bowing.
5   Sarcomatous change.

Stems

A   Paget's disease.
B   Osteogenesis Imperfecta.
C   Rickets.
D   Osteomalacia.
E   Osteoporosis.

Question 17. Osteomyelitis

Choose the pathogens most commonly related to the following conditions.

Options

1   *Salmonella.*
2   *Pseudomonas aeruginosa.*
3   *Staphylococcus aureus.*
4   *Haemophilus influenzae.*
5   *Eikenella corrodens.*

Stems

A   Teenager wearing trainers who has stepped on a nail and has a web space infection of the foot.
B   Rugby player with an infected second MCPJ after hitting another player in a lineout.
C   18-month-old girl with temperature, rigors, and a limp.
D   Sickle-cell disease.
E   Infected non-union open distal tibial fracture in a 32-year-old man.

Question 18. Bone tumours

Options

1   8-year-old boy with vertebra plana and no soft tissue mass on MRI.
2   12-year-old boy with painless well-marginated lucent lesion in the proximal metaphysic of the humerus.
3   15-year-old boy with knee pain at night and a poorly defined femoral diaphyseal lesion radiographically with an associated soft tissue mass.
4   66-year-old man with groin pain and an ill-defined lesion of the iliac wing with calcification within it on AP of the pelvis.
5   22-year-old woman with 2mm CT proven lesion with central nidus in the lesser trochanter, pain alleviated by NSAIDs at night.

Stems

A   Chondrosarcoma.
B   Ewings sarcoma.
C   Unicameral bone cyst.
D   Langerhans Cell Histiocytosis X (Eosinophilic granuloma).
E   Osteoid osteoma.

Question 19. Dupuytren's disease

For each of the clinical scenarios choose the most appropriate operation.

Options

1   Dermofasciectomy combined with full-thickness skin grafting.
2   Limited fasciectomy.
3   Subcutaneous fasciotomy.
4   Amputation of digit.

Stems

A   Dupuytren's diathesis.
B   Elderly patient with 20-degree contracture of MCPJ and co-existent multiple morbidity.
C   Multiply operated digit with recurrent 90-degree fixed contracture of the proximal interphalangeal joint (PIPJ) and vascular compromise.
D   Previously operated digit with recurring contracture.
E   Early presentation with 20-degree contracture MCPJ in a 54-year-old epileptic man.

Question 20. Orthopaedic appliances

Select the most appropriate appliance/s for assisting in the management of the following conditions.

Options

1   Lively splint.
2   Ankle foot orthosis.
3   Abduction brace.
4   University of California Berkeley Laborotary type orthosis.
5   Boston brace.

Stems

A   Developmental dysplasia of the hip.
B   Cerebral palsy.
C   Tibialis posterior dysfunction.
D   Scoliosis.
E   Radial nerve palsy.

Answer 1   A3, B1 & 4, C1 & 2, D2, E5

Taurus fractures are stable fractures. Displaced epiphyseal fractures need reducing to reduce the risk of growth plate arrest. Unstable Colles' fractures need reducing and more often than not k-wires are needed to hold the reduction. Smith's fractures are very difficult to control with POP alone. Colles' and Smith's fractures are 'fragility' fractures, so osteoporosis must be considered. A Galleazi fracture in an adult needs to be taken to theatre for plating of the radius and screening of the DRUJ. If this is unstable, then its reduction can be held with either k-wires or a screw.

Answer 2   A2, B5, C4, D3, E1

A displaced fracture in anyone under 60 is an emergency. If a sub-capital fracture is not too displaced then manipulation and reduction with cannulated screw fixation is an option, although there is still a significant chance of avascular necrosis. Displaced sub-capital fractures are usually treated with a hemiarthroplasty. A bi-polar implant is considered in younger or more active patients in an effort to decrease acetabular wear. The majority of inter-trochanteric fractures are amenable to reduction and fixation with a DHS.

Answer 3   A2, B1, C3, D5, E4

There is a very high chance (50%) of popliteal artery damage with a dislocated knee and this must be investigated and treated as soon as possible. Acute dislocations of the patella are traditionally treated in an above knee pop but there is a move to more aggressive treatment with repair of the medial patello-femoral ligament in some centres. Swelling within 2 hours of an injury usually represents a haemarthrosis. The commonest causes are fracture, ruptured anterior cruciate ligament (ACL) and peripheral meniscal tears. With a large valgus force to the knee, the medial collateral ligament (MCL), the medial meniscus and the ACL can be damaged (O'Donaghue's triad). The MCL can be managed non-operatively in a brace, but operative intervention can be considered for the meniscus and ACL, after the MCL has healed.

Answer 4   A1, B3, C4, D2, E5

Young gymnasts, athletes and fast bowlers are prone to pars defects. Night pain and sweats are a couple of 'Red Flag' symptoms; malignancy and infection must be ruled out. Back pain in young children must be investigated to rule out infection and tumours. Back pain and sudden urinary incontinence is indicative of a 'Cauda Equina' syndrome which needs rapid investigation and surgical decompression of the offending compressive lesion. Chronic low back pain is a common problem; the majority of patients can be treated conservatively.

Answer 5   A1, 3, 4 & 5, B2, 3, 4 & 5, C1 & 3, D1 & 4, E3 & 5

Septic arthritis is an orthopaedic emergency. Diagnosis can be difficult in immunocomprimised patients, patients on ITU, and in either the very young or very old. A high index of suspicion and the presence of organisms on microscopy or gram stain forms an essential part of the diagnosis. The treatment is surgical and may require repeat visits to theatre.

Answer 6   A3, B6, C1 & 5, D2, E4

The Gustilo & Anderson classification of open fractures relates to the severity of the injury in terms of the velocity of the mechanism and the degree of soft-tissue damage.

Type I   1cm wound or less, low energy.
Type II   >1cm wound with moderate soft-tissue damage.
Type III   Extensive soft-tissue damage, crush injuries due to high velocity trauma and subdivided into:

    III a: Adequate soft tissue coverage and bone cover.
    III b: Bone is exposed together with periosteal stripping.
    III c: Any open fracture where there is vascular impairment.

Answer 7   A5 & 6, B3, C4, D2, E1

Compartment syndrome is a combination of signs and symptoms that result from increased pressure within a confined space. There are a variety of possible aetiologies; they can be extrinsic, such as dressings and plasters, as well as intrinsic such as haemorrhage from fractures (including open fractures) and oedema related to anaphylaxis (snake bite for example). Burns are an important cause that is often forgotten; when circumferential to an area or extremity, escharotomy is often required.

Answer 8   A4, B2 & 3, C6, D1 & 5

A number of fractures are more commonly known by their eponyms. Knowledge of fracture eponyms aids accurate description and communication between professionals.

Answer 9   A3, B5, C1, D2, E4

Fracture classification systems are used in orthopaedics and trauma to aid in offering a prognosis for fracture patterns that can be commonly grouped together within regions. The AO classification system is a universal system that can be applied to any long bone. Knowledge of classification systems aids accurate fracture description and communication between professionals, as well as allowing for comparison of treatment methods in research.

Answer 10   A3 & 4, B none, C1, D2, E4

Answer 11   A1, B3 & 5, C2 & 5, D4 & 5, E5

Hinged knees are highly constrained and can cause mechanical loosening. They should be used only for low demand patients requiring a revision or where there is severe pre-operative deformity/instability. Unicompartmental knee replacement requires the presence of the ACL to provide stability, as the prosthesis is unable to provide inherent stability. The results of both fixed bearing, mobile bearing and unicompartmental knee replacement are very good at 10 years plus in the published literature.

Answer 12   A5, B4, C1, D2, E3

Answer 13   A1 & 3, B1 & 5, C1, D1 & 2, E1 & 4

Answer 14   A5, B1, C4, D3, E2

It is probably worth trying footwear modification with most of the above patients initially. It is important to get weight-bearing x-rays and measure the hallux valgus angle and the intermetatarsal angle as these help in deciding the type of operation that can be offered. The condition of the 1st MTPJ is also important. If degenerate, then fusion of the joint or arthroplasty (either hemi or total) will be required.

Answer 15   A1, 2 & 3, B1, 2, 3 & 4, C1, 2 & 3, D1 & 2, E4

The causes of a limp are numerous in childhood. Referred pain must be remembered and knee pain is often a cardinal sign of hip pathology and even spine pathology (eg. discitis). Osgood Schlatter's disease is a traction apophysitis and can almost be considered physiological in terms of its common nature and age of presentation (adolescent growth spurt usually). The possibility of NAI (Non-Accidental Injury) must always be borne in mind when dealing with children.

Answer 16   A1, 3, 4 & 5, B1, 3 & 4, C1, 2, 3 & 4, D1, 3 & 4, E2 & 3

Looser's zones are also known as pseudofractures and can be found in a number of disorders. A pathological fracture occurs through an area of abnormal bone and often therefore requires little force. Up to 5% of patients with longstanding Paget's disease are at risk of malignant change.

Answer 17   A2 & 3, B3 & 5, C2, 3 & 4, D1 & 3, E3

Staphylococcus aureus is the commonest bone infection pathogen. Young children are prone also to a number of other pathogens including *Haemophilus influenza* and *Pseudomonas aeruginosa*. Sickle-cell disease is often associated with Salmonella. Human 'fight bites' at the MCPJs are notoriously overlooked and for the most part should be explored and the wound left open.

Answer 18   A4, B3, C2, D1, E5

The differential diagnosis of vertebra plana includes osteosarcoma; a soft-tissue mass is usually present in such rare cases. Age and site presentation are important in the differential diagnosis of bone tumours. Enneking's questions relate to the site, to what the bone is doing to the tumour, to what the tumour is doing to the bone, and to whether there is any soft tissue or distant spread.

Answer 19   A1, B3, C4, D1, E2

Dupuytren's diathesis is an aggressive and severe form of the disease that occurs at an early age. It is usually associated with a family history, knuckle pads, plantar (Ledderhosen's disease) and penile (Peyronie's disease) fibromatosis. Subcutaneous fasciotomy is a minimal procedure, usually under local anaesthetic and reserved for the elderly or where extensive surgery may be contraindicated.

Answer 20   A3, B2 & 3, (1), C4, D5, E1

Orthotics are used for support and maintain limb or body part positions. They will hopefully prevent progression of disorders and enable improved function in the presence of an abnormality. Prosthetics improve function by replacing missing parts.

Chapter 13

Burns & plastic surgery

Peter Drew, MB BCh (Wales) FRCS (Eng) FRCS (Ed) FRCS (Plast)
Consultant in Plastic and Reconstructive Surgery
Morriston Hospital, Swansea, UK

For all questions each option may be used once, more than once or not at all.

Question 1. Wound healing

Match each of the following stems with the appropriate phase or clinical type of wound healing listed in the options.

Options

1   Remodelling.
2   Delayed primary closure.
3   Healing by secondary intension.
4   Cellular proliferation and extra-cellular matrix deposition.
5   Healing by primary intension.
6   Inflammation.

Stems

A   Healing by granulation and contraction.
B   The phase of wound healing characterized by the appearance of macrophages in a wound.
C   Closure of a wound several days following an initial debridement.
D   The phase of wound healing characterized by the appearance of fibroblasts in a wound.

Question 2. Skin

Match the following cell types and structures with the most appropriate description of their position or function.

Options

1 Keratinocyte.
2 Melanocyte.
3 Langerhans' cell.
4 Merkel cell.
5 Fibroblast.
6 Pacinian corpuscle.
7 Myofibroblast.

Stems

A The cell type responsible for wound contraction.
B A dendritic cell found in the basal layers of the epidermis.
C A collagen-producing cell found in the dermis.
D The main cell type found in the epidermis.
E A cell type producing protection from ultra-violet light.

Question 3. Upper limb pathology

Match the following acronyms with the most appropriate description of a clinical sign, condition or disease affecting the upper limb.

Options

1 Garrod.
2 Fromet.
3 Phalen.
4 Poland.
5 Heberden.

Stems

A   A clinical sign associated with Dupuytren's disease.
B   A clinical test used to diagnose median nerve compression at the wrist.
C   Deformity at the distal interphalangeal joint in osteoarthritis.
D   A syndrome which may include deformity of the chest wall or cardiovascular system with upper limb abnormality.
E   A clinical sign seen when adductor pollicis is non-functional.

Question 4. Upper limb anatomy

Match the following major nerves in the upper limb with the most appropriate description of nerve type, distribution or function.

Options

1   Median nerve.
2   Ulnar nerve.
3   Radial nerve.
4   Posterior interosseous nerve.
5   Musculocutaneous nerve.

Stems

A   A mixed (motor and sensory) nerve that innervates Triceps and gives sensation to the area on the dorsum of the 1st web space.
B   A mixed (motor and sensory) nerve that innervates Biceps and gives sensation to the posterior-lateral forearm.
C   A mixed (motor and sensory) nerve that innervates extensor pollicis longus.
D   A mixed (motor and sensory) nerve that innervates two lumbricals and abductor pollicis brevis.
E   A mixed (motor and sensory) nerve that innervates two lumbricals and adductor pollicis.

Question 5. Skin grafts

Match the following clinical scenarios with the most appropriate method of wound closure.

Options

1   Meshed partial (split) thickness skin graft.
2   Unmeshed partial (split) thickness skin graft.
3   Full-thickness skin graft.
4   Z plasty.

Stems

A   A 1.5cm diameter skin defect at the medial canthus following excision of a BCC in a 70-year-old man.
B   A 15 x 10cm defect on the lower leg following burn excision in a 50-year-old man.
C   A 7 x 5cm defect on the dorsum of the hand following burn excision in a 19-year-old female.
D   Small defects on the fingers following syndactyly release in a 1-year-old boy.

Question 6. Skin transplantation

Match the following stems and options.

Options

1   Allograft.
2   Isograft.
3   Xenograft.
4   Autograft.

Stems

A   Skin taken from the recipient.
B   Skin taken from a genetically different individual of the same species as the recipient.
C   Skin taken from a genetically identical individual of the same species as the recipient (i.e. an identical twin).
D   Skin taken from an individual of a different species to the recipient.

Question 7. Skin flaps

Match the following types of local skin flap with the most appropriate description of flap design or function.

Options

1 Rotation flap.
2 Transposition flap.
3 Advancement flap.
4 Axial pattern flap.
5 Random pattern flap.

Stems

A   A skin flap designed without specific vessels running longitudinally within it.
B   A skin flap designed to move in an arc around a pivot point, to fill an adjacent defect.
C   A skin flap designed to move forward to fill an adjacent defect, without lateral movement.
D   A skin flap designed with a specific vessel running longitudinally within it.
E   A skin flap designed to move laterally about a pivot point to fill an adjacent defect.

Question 8. Burn resuscitation

You are managing the fluid resuscitation of a 75kg adult patient with 40% total body surface area (TBSA) burns, using Hartmann's solution given according to the formula (4ml/kg/%TBSA). Select the most appropriate option for each of the following stems.

Options

1   0.5ml.
2   6000mls.
3   375mls.
4   5-10mls.
5   5625mls.

Stems

A   The estimated total volume of Hartmann's solution required during the 8-hour period from the time of the burn.
B   The lowest acceptable hourly urine output per kg body weight.
C   The estimated hourly volume of Hartmann's solution required during the period from 8 to 24 hours after the burn.
D   The volume of additional Hartmann's solution per kg body weight given as a bolus if urine output dips below an acceptable level.
E   The patient's estimated blood volume.

Question 9. Burns

Match the following descriptions of burn injuries with the most likely clinical scenarios.

Options

1   A deep dermal (deep partial-thickness) burn.
2   A superficial partial-thickness burn.
3   A high-voltage electrical burn.
4   A low-voltage electrical burn.
5   An acid burn.
6   An alkali burn.

Stems

A   A painful, black burn with a slimy appearance, testing positive
    when red litmus paper is applied.
B   A brick-red burn with a fixed, non-blanching mottled appearance.
C   A bright pink, blanching burn with a moist surface and blisters.
D   A very deep, charred burn in the palm of a man with a painful,
    swollen forearm and a similar burn on his foot.
E   Pain under the fingernail in a man brought in from his place of
    work.
F   A man with painful burns on his knees following a day spent laying
    concrete.

Question 10. Burns - surface area estimation

Match the following stems with the most likely estimate of % total body
surface area (TBSA).

Options

1   1% TBSA.
2   9% TBSA.
3   18% TBSA.
4   36% TBSA.
5   46% TBSA.

Stems

A   The approximate % TBSA of the head and neck in an adult.
B   The approximate % TBSA of the head and neck in a 1-year-old
    child.
C   The approximate % TBSA of an arm in an adult.
D   The approximate % TBSA of both lower limbs (including the
    buttocks, genitals and perineum) in an adult.
E   The approximate % TBSA of both lower limbs (including the
    buttocks, genitals and perineum) in a 1-year-old child.

Question 11. Malignant melanoma

Match the following.

Options

1   Lentigo Maligna Melanoma.
2   Superficial Spreading Melanoma.
3   Acral Lentiginous Melanoma.
4   Nodular Melanoma.
5   Lentigo Maligna.
6   Subungal Melanoma.

Stems

A   The commonest type of malignant melanoma.
B   A sub-type of melanoma commonly misdiagnosed initially as a traumatic or fungal lesion.
C   Typically presents as a nodule or darkened area within a long-standing pigmented lesion on the face of an elderly farmer.
D   The type of melanoma which makes up a much higher proportion of tumours seen in dark-skinned races than in Caucasians.
E   A melanoma exhibiting a greater vertical than horizontal growth phase.

Question 12. Malignant melanoma

Match the following.

Options

1   Breslow thicknes 0.5mm, Clark level 1.
2   Breslow thickness 1.4mm, Clark level 2.
3   Breslow thickness 2.1mm, Clark level 3.
4   Breslow thickness 3mm, Clark level 4.
5   Breslow thickness 4.3mm, Clark level 5.

Stems

A   A nodular melanoma invading the reticular dermis.
B   A superficial spreading melanoma invading to the papillary-reticular junction.
C   A nodular melanoma invading the sub-cuticular fat.
D   A Lentigo Maligna Melanoma.

Question 13. Skin cancer

Match the following.

Options

1   Bowen's disease.
2   Solar keratosis
3   Basal Cell Carcinoma (BCC).
4   Squamous Cell Carcinoma (SCC).
5   Keratoacanthoma.
6   Seborrhoeic keratosis.

Stems

A   A rapidly growing lesion on the face of an elderly man, which has a central 'plug' of keratin and eventually resolves spontaneously.
B   A hyperkeratotic patch on the leg of an elderly lady. Histology shows intra-epidermal carcinoma.
C   A 2cm diameter ulcerating lesion with an everted edge on the lower leg of a patient taking immunosuppressive medication.
D   Multiple keratoses on the scalp and face of a bald WW2 veteran.
E   A 1cm diameter raised lesion with a 'pearly' edge and telangectasia.

Question 14. Cleft lip and palate

The following relate to the usual timing of various surgical procedures in an otherwise normal child born with a complete unilateral cleft lip and palate.

Options

1   3 months.
2   5-7 years.
3   9-12 months.
4   9 years.
5   16 years.

Stems

A   Alveolar bone graft.
B   Cleft palate repair.
C   Pharyngoplasty.
D   Rhinoplasty.
E   Cleft lip repair.

Question 15. Local anaesthesia

You are operating on a 70kg patient under local anaesthesia. The only available agents are 1% Lignocaine (either plain or with 1 in 200,000 Adrenaline) and plain 0.25% Bupivocaine.

Options

1   49mls.
2   56mls.
3   200mls.
4   28mls.

Stems

A   The maximum dose of plain Lignocaine.

B   The maximum dose of Bupivocaine.

C   The maximum dose of Lignocaine with Adrenaline 1 in 200,000.

D   The volume in which 1ml of 1:1000 Adrenaline should be diluted to give a 1 in 200,000 solution.

Answer 1   A3, B6, C2, D4

Broadly speaking, the molecular and cellular biology of wound healing can be considered to proceed through three consecutive (but not mutually exclusive) stages, i.e. inflammation, cellular proliferation/extra-cellular matrix deposition and remodelling. Macrophages are an essential feature of the inflammatory phase, while fibroblasts characterize the phase of cellular proliferation/extra-cellular matrix deposition. Clinically, wound healing is described as occurring by primary closure, (i.e. immediate suture), delayed primary closure, (i.e. initial cleaning and debridement followed by closure after a period of days) and healing by secondary intension, (i.e. by granulation and contraction).

Answer 2   A7, B2, C5, D1, E2

The epidermis is predominantly composed of keratinocytes progressing from the basal layer outward, to be shed as squams. Melanocytes are dendritic cells seen in the basal layer of the epidermis, with intracellular attachments to numerous basal keratinocytes. Melanocytes produce and export melanin, a protein conveying protection from UV light. Fibroblasts are the predominant cell type found in the dermis, the main function of which is collagen synthesis. A variant, the myofibroblast, is responsible for wound contraction.

Answer 3   A1, B3, C5, D4, E2

Garrod's knuckle pads are thickenings of the subcutaneous tissue over the extensor side of the proximal interphalangeal joints, seen in around 20% of cases of Dupuytren's disease. Fromet's sign is positive when paralysis of adductor pollicis requires the patient to flex the interphalageal joint of the thumb (flexor pollicis longus) to enable him to grip a piece of paper placed in the first web space. The ulnar nerve innervates adductor pollicis. Phalen's test is used to diagnose carpal tunnel syndrome, while Heberden's nodes are deformities caused by osteoarthritic osteophytes at the distal interphalagael joints. Poland's syndrome is a rare birth defect which may include abnormalities of the upper limb and chest.

References and further reading
1.   Lister G. *The Hand. Diagnosis and Indications*. Churchill Livingstone, Edinburgh, 1984.

Answer 4   A3, B5, C3, D1, E2

Self-explanantory.

References and further reading
1.   On behalf of the Guarantors of Brain. *Aids to the examination of the peripheral nervous system.* Bailliere Tindall, London, 1986.

Answer 5   A3, B1, C2, D3

Small defects in anatomical areas where cosmesis is important (eg.the face) are best dealt with using full-thickness skin taken from the same anatomical region (eg. post-auricular skin). Full-thickness skin is also the most appropriate option when it is important to avoid post-graft contraction, for example in a child's hands. Larger defects in non-exposed areas are best grafted using a meshed partial-thickness skin graft, while an unmeshed graft is more appropriate in exposed areas.

References and further reading
1.   McGregor AD, McGregor IJ. *Fundamental Techniques of Plastic Surgery.* 9th Edition. Churchill Livingstone, London, 1995.

Answer 6   A4, B1, C2, D3

Self-explanatory.

Answer 7   A5, B1, C3, D4, E2

Self-explanatory.

References and further reading
1.   McGregor AD, McGregor IJ. *Fundamental Techniques of Plastic Surgery.* 9th Edition. Churchill Livingstone, London, 1995.

Answer 8   A2, B1, C3, D4, E5

The Parkland formula estimates the volume of Hartmann's solution required over the first 24 hours from the time of a burn injury of = 15% TBSA in an adult. Half the calculated volume is given over the first 8 hours and half over the subsequent 16 hours. Clinical indicators of intravascular volume (i.e. pulse, BP, CVP, urine output, etc.) are assessed regularly during resuscitation. An hourly urine output of <0.5mls/kg in an adult should prompt a more detailed appraisal and an additional bolus of 5-10mls/kg Hartmann's solution in the first instance.

References and further reading
1.   SA Pape, K Judkins, JAD Settle. *Burns - The first five days.* 2nd edition. Smith & Nephew, 2001
2.   Emergency Management of Severe Burns (EMSB) Provider Manual, 1996.

Answer 9   A6, B1, C2, D3, E5, F6

A blistered burn with a moist, pink-looking bed which blanches is usually a superficial partial thickness injury, i.e. injury to the mid-dermal level. A red looking, mottled burn which does not blanch, however, is likely to be deep partial thickness (deep dermal).

High voltage electrical injury may produce deep entry and exit wounds at sites far distant from each other. Current transmission through the intervening tissues may produce tissue necrosis, commonly manifesting as compartment syndrome in the limbs.

Both acid and alkali burns may be painful while the chemical agent concerned remains on the skin in high concentration. Treatment is thus aimed at diluting the chemical and physically removing it by copious irrigation with water. Pain beneath the fingernails is a frequent finding in incompletely treated acid burns on the hands. Calcium gluconate gel is supplied as first-aid for burns from hydrofluoric acid. Strong alkali (eg. caustic soda) reacts with fat in tissues to produce 'soap' (saponification) giving such injuries a slimy appearance. Lime in cement is a common source of alkali burns.

Answer 9   contd:-

References and further reading
1. SA Pape, K Judkins, JAD Settle. *Burns - The first five days.* 2nd edition. Smith & Nephew, 2001.
2. Emeregency Management of Severe Burns (EMSB) Provider Manual, 1996
3. D Herndon, Ed. *Total Burn Care.* 2nd edition. WB Saunders London, 2002
4. JAD Settle. *Principles and Practice of Burns Management.* Churchill Livingstone, London, 1996.

Answer 10   A2, B3, C2, D5, E4

Lund & Broder charts are widely available and when properly used, can give an accurate estimation of the % of the total body surface area affected by a burn injury. When not available, the 'rule of nines' gives an easily remembered alternative.

Body proportions change with age. The proportion of the total surface area represented by the head of a neonate is around double that of an adult, while the lower limbs make up a smaller proportion than in the adult.

References and further reading
1. SA Pape, K Judkins, JAD Settle. *Burns - The first five days.* 2nd edition. Smith & Nephew, 2001.
2. Emergency Management of Severe Burns (EMSB) Provider Manual, 1996.
3. D Herndon, Ed. *Total Burn Care.* 2nd edition. WB Saunders London, 2002
4. JAD Settle. *Principles and Practice of Burns Management.* Churchill Livingstone, London, 1996.

Answer 11   A2, B6, C1, D3, E4

Self-explanatory.

Answer 12   A4, B3, C5, D1

Clark levels describe various levels of invasion of the skin, while Breslow thickness is the maximum thickness of the tumour measured from the stratum granulosum in the epidermis. Tumour thickness has some prognostic value.

Answer 13   A5, B1, C4, D2, E3

Answer 14   A4, B3, C2, D5, E1

Answer 15   A4, B2, C1, D3

The maximum dose of Lignocaine is 4mg/kg plain or 7mg/kg with adrenaline. Adrenaline has the effect of prolonging the action of the local anaesthetic by delaying systemic absorption. The maximum dose of Bupivocaine (plain or with adrenaline) is 2mg/kg.

References and further reading
   1.   BNF.

Chapter 14
Ear, nose & throat surgery

Mriganka De, MRCS (Ed) MRCS (Glas)
Specialist Registrar, Otolaryngology, West Midlands Rotation, UK
Yogesh Bajaj, MS MRCS (Ed)
Research Fellow, Otolaryngology, Great Ormond Street, London, UK

For all questions each option may be used once, more than once or not at all.

Question 1. Hearing loss

Options

1   Waardenburg's syndrome.
2   Pendred's syndrome.
3   Glue ear.
4   Mal development of cochlear.

Stems

A   3½-year-old child with fluctuating hearing loss.
B   Rudimentary pinna with hearing loss.
C   Sensorineural hearing loss with goitre.
D   Eyelid deformity, deep blue eyes with hearing loss.

Question 2. Stridor

Options

1 Foreign body.
2 Epiglottitis.
3 Laryngomalacia.
4 Laryngeal papillomatosis.

Stems

A 5-year-old child with fever, drooling of saliva and stridor.
B Sudden onset stridor in an otherwise normal child.
C Intermittent stridor in a newborn child.
D Stridor with hoarseness of voice.

Question 3. Neck lumps (child)

Options

1 Sebaceous cyst.
2 Cystic hygroma.
3 Infected branchial cyst.
4 Thyroglossal cyst.

Stems

A Midline swelling moves with tongue protrusion and swallowing.
B Bluish translucent neck swelling in a child.
C Painful swelling in the anterior triangle of the neck in a teenager.
D 12-year-old with posterior triangle swelling with a punctum.

Question 4. Nasal obstruction

Options

1 Choanal atresia.
2 Inverted papilloma.
3 Angiofibroma.
4 Foreign body.
5 Cystic fibrosis.

Stems

A   Unilateral nasal obstruction with bleeding.
B   Nasal obstruction with bronchiectasis and nasal polyposis.
C   Nasal obstruction in a newborn child.
D   Nasal obstruction with large nasal polyp.
E   Unilateral foul swelling, nasal discharge.

Question 5. Dysphagia

Options

1 Post-cricoid cancer.
2 Bulbar palsy.
3 Food bolus obstruction.
4 Pharyngeal pouch.
5 Plummer Vinson syndrome.

Stems

A   Elderly female with known Alzheimer dementia and dysphagia.
B   Elderly male with dysphagia associated with regurgitation of undigested food.
C   Dysphagia associated with koilonychia anaemia.
D   Middle-aged male with chronic alcoholism and dysphagia.
E   Elderly with recent severe dysphagia.

Question 6. Neck lump (adult)

Options

1   Hodgkin's lymphoma.
2   Hypopharyngeal cancer.
3   Laryngocele.
4   Glandular fever.

Stems

A   60-year-old heavy smoker with a sore throat.
B   40-year-old lady with bilateral rubbery nodes with night sweats.
C   A young man with fever, sore throat and lymphocytosis.
D   50-year-old male with intermittent neck swelling, becomes prominent on Valsalva's manoeuvre.

Question 7. Sore throat

Options

1   Tonsilliar malignancy.
2   Quinsy.
3   Reflux.
4   Acute tonsillitis.

Stems

A   Young man with fever and sore throat.
B   Elderly gentleman, heavy smoker with sore throat.
C   Young patient with fever and trismus and sore throat.
D   Anxious young, obese female with sore throat.

Question 8. Hoarseness of voice

Options

1   Vocal cord nodule.
2   Laryngeal cancer.
3   Chronic sinusitis.
4   Reinke's oedema.

Stems

A   Recent onset hoarseness of voice in a 60-year-old man who smokes 22-30 cigarettes a day.
B   40-year-old teacher with hoarseness.
C   Middle-aged lady with hoarseness and hypothyroidism.
D   Intermittent hoarseness, cough and postnasal drip.

Question 9. Salivary gland tumours

Options

1   Keratoconjunctivitis sicca syndrome.
2   Pleomorphic adenoma.
3   Adenocystic carcinoma.
4   Mumps.
5   Duct calculus.

Stems

A   20-year-old female with right submandibular swelling related to food.
B   5-year-old boy with inflamed tender parotid swelling.
C   Unilateral slow-growing tumour in a middle-aged male.
D   Rapidly growing submandibular gland tumour with pain radiating to face and occiput.
E   Bilateral submandibular and parotid hyperthrophy with dry eyes and mouth.

Question 10. Thyroid

Options

1   Endemic goitre.
2   Medullary carcinoma.
3   Anaplastic carcinoma.
4   Hashimoto's thyroiditis.
5   Toxic nodular goitre.

Stems

A   25-year-old female with midline neck swelling, palpitation, tremor.
B   30-year-old female with tiredness and thyroid enlargement.
C   49-year-old female with tender midline neck swelling with raised thyroxin levels.
D   85-year-old gentleman with rapidly growing thyroid lump.
E   Middle-aged male with hypotension, hypercalcaemia and thyroid swelling.

Question 11. Tinnitus

Options

1   Presbycusis.
2   Menière's disease.
3   Glomus jugulare.
4   Acoustic neuroma.

Stems

A   Unilateral tinnitus with asymmetrical hearing loss.
B   Bilateral tinnitus in an elderly male.
C   Tinnitus deafness and vertigo in a young female.
D   Middle-aged man with pulsatile tinnitus and *sunrise* sign on otoscopy.

Question 12. Vertigo

Options

1 Vestibular neuronitis.
2 Benign positional vertigo.
3 Perilymphatic fistula.
4 Vertebrobasilar insufficiency.

Stems

A Vertigo associated with particular head movements lasting for a few seconds.
B Vertigo associated with lower cranial nerve palsy.
C Vertigo lasting for weeks associated with hearing loss preceded by upper respiratory tract infection.
D Vertigo following mastoid surgery.

Question 13. Facial palsy

Options

1 Ramsey Hunt syndrome.
2 Bell's palsy.
3 Cholesteatoma.
4 Temporal bone fracture.

Stems

A Lower motor neurone palsy of acute onset in a middle-aged man with normal hearing.
B Facial palsy associated with otorrhoea.
C Facial palsy after head injury.
D Facial palsy associated with blisters in the ear canal.

Question 14. Otorrhoea

Options

1 Malignant otitis externa.
2 Mastoiditis.
3 Otitis externa.
4 Cholesteatoma.
5 Otitis media.

Stems

A 20-year-old male with discharging ear and eczema.
B 40-year-old diabetic female with severe ear ache.
C Otorrhoea in a 2-year-old child with upper respiratory tract infection.
D Otorrhoea associated with polyp in the ear canal.
E Otorrhoea associated with post-aural swelling.

Question 15. Earache

Options

1 Temporomandibular joint (TMJ) dysfunction.
2 Eustachian tube dysfunction.
3 Impacted wax.
4 Perichondritis.
5 Bullous myringitis.

Stems

A Elderly female using hearing aid with earache.
B Young male with swollen pinna.
C Middle-aged gentleman with blisters in tympanic membrane.
D Young female with crepitation of TMJ.
E Young male complaining of earache with normal ear drum.

Question 16. Ear operation

Options

1   Endolypmphatic sac decompression.
2   Stapedectomy.
3   Myringoplasty.
4   Myringotomy.
5   Mastoidectomy.

Stems

A   Perforated ear drum.
B   Cholesteatoma.
C   Menière's disease.
D   Otosclerosis.
E   Glue ear.

Question 17. Hearing loss

Options

1   Glue ear.
2   Otosclerosis.
3   Noise-induced hearing loss.
4   Drug-induced hearing loss.
5   Nasopharyngeal tumour.
6   Presbycusis.

Stems

A   Elderly gentleman with hearing loss and tinnitus.
B   Middle-aged gentleman with conductive hearing loss and nasal obstruction.
C   Young child with hearing loss and dull tympanic membrane.
D   Young female with bilateral conductive hearing loss.
E   Middle-aged man with hearing loss and past history of working in Armed Forces.
F   Elderly female who was treated in the past with Gentamycin for chest infection.

Question 18. Nasal obstruction

Options

1   Choanal atresia.
2   Sinusitis.
3   Septal haematoma.
4   Rhinitis.
5   Inverted papilloma.

Stems

A   Nasal obstruction in a middle-aged man with rhinorrhoea.
B   Nasal obstruction associated with unilateral nasal polyp.
C   Nasal obstruction in a newborn child.
D   Foul-smelling nasal discharge in a 40-year-old.
E   Nasal obstruction following nasal trauma.

Question 19. Epistaxis

Options

1   Warfarin-induced.
2   Metastatic.
3   Hereditary haemorrhagic telangiectasia.
4   Sinonasal tumour.

Stems

A   Elderly gentleman with nosebleed and right-sided nasal obstruction.
B   Elderly female with known atrial fibrillation.
C   60-year-old gentleman with renal cell carcinoma.
D   25-year-old gentleman with red spots on lips, mucous membranes of the tongue and mouth.

Question 20. Facial pain

Options

1   Migraine.
2   Post-herpetic neuralgia.
3   Chronic sinusitis.
4   Trigeminal neuralgia.

Stems

A   Facial pain associated with purulent nasal discharge.
B   Unilateral facial pain with aura in 40-year-old female.
C   Unilateral intensive facial pain as the trigger point.
D   Facial pain with the vesicles in the face.

Question 21. Rhinorrhoea

Options

1   CSF rhinorrhoea.
2   Chronic sinusitis.
3   Bilateral nasal polyp.
4   Allergic rhinitis.

Stems

A   Bilateral nasal obstruction.
B   Rhinorrhoea with seasonal variations.
C   Rhinorrhoea following head injury.
D   Rhinorrhoea in a poorly controlled diabetic.

Question 22. Nasal polyposis

Options

1   Sinonasal malignancy.
2   Antrochoanal polyp.
3   Treatment of choice is functional endoscopic sinus surgery.
4   Cystic fibrosis.

Stems

A   Nasal polyp associated with bronchiectasis in a young child.
B   Unilateral polyp bleeds on touch.
C   Young adult with unilateral nasal obstruction.
D   Recurrent nasal polyposis.

Answer 1   A3, B4, C2, D1

Glue ear (otitis media with effusion) is a common condition affecting children under 5 years of age. The fluid in the middle ear keeps appearing (along with colds) and disappearing; as a result, the child has fluctuating deafness.

Rudimentary pinna (microtia) is usually associated with inner ear and middle ear anomalies causing conductive, sensorineural or mixed hearing loss.

Pendred's syndrome is an autosomal recessive trait characterised by severe sensorineural hearing loss, enlarged goitre and hypothyroidism in a child.

Waardenburg's syndrome is an autosomal dominant trait characterised by white forelock, different colour of iris and lateral displacement of medial canthi.

Answer 2   A2, B1, C3, D4

Acute epiglottitis is caused by *Haemophilus influenzae* in the majority of cases. It commonly occurs from 3 to 6 years of age. The common presentation is a fit child complaining of a sore throat which progresses to dysphagia within half an hour and stridor within 2 hours.

Foreign body inhalation has a typical history of a normal child who suddenly develops a violent bout of cough while playing with small toys or eating peanuts. The child may then develop stridor or respiratory distress depending on the position of the foreign body.

Laryngomalacia is the most common cause of congenital stridor. It is characterised by flaccidity of supraglottic structures. The stridor is intermittent and reaches a maximum between 9-12 months and then begins to resolve.

Laryngeal papillomatosis is caused by a DNA virus of the papova group. The papillomas can be present anywhere in the larynx and the trachea. The management depends on the extent of the infection and airway obstruction.

Answer 3   A4, B2, C3, D1

A thyroglossal cyst is a remnant of the thyroglossal tract (along which the thyroid gland descends into the neck from the tongue base). The recommended treatment is Sistrunk's operation, i.e. removal of all the tract remnants along with the central part of the hyoid bone.

A cystic hygroma is a unilocular or multilocular lymphangioma, which is usually slow-growing. Surgery is the mainstay of treatment.

A branchial cyst is a developmental anomaly of the second branchial cleft. The usual site is at the junction of upper 2/3 and lower 1/3 of the anterior border of the sternomastoid. The treatment is surgical excision.

A sebaceous cyst is a well-encapsulated collection of sebum as a result of the blockage of the duct of the sebaceous gland. The overlying skin is tethered to the cyst. It pits on pressure (Pitting sign) because of its contents.

Answer 4   A3, B5, C1, D2, E4

Angiofibroma is a vascular swelling presenting in the nasopharynx of adolescent males. Nasal obstruction and bleeding are the cardinal symptoms. The treatment is surgical excision.

Cystic fibrosis is an autosomal recessive multisystem disease. The systems mostly affected are the respiratory and digestive tract. High levels of sodium in the sweat is diagnostic.

Choanal atresia is a congenital abnormality resulting from failure of canalisation of the posterior nasal cavities. Bilateral atresia presents as a respiratory emergency as the newborn is an obligate nasal breather. The treatment is surgical correction.

Inverted papilloma is seen in 50-60-year-olds. It is characterised by a polypoidal lesion arising from the lateral nasal wall. The treatment is surgical excision with close follow-up.

Nasal foreign bodies are characterised by nasal obstruction and a foul-smelling nasal discharge which is unilateral. The treatment is removal of the foreign body and antibiotics.

Answer 5   A3, B4, C5, D1, E2

Patients with food bolus obstruction are usually elderly patients who are not able to chew the food very well, with maybe an underlying oesophageal stricture. The patient presents with drooling (inability to swallow his own saliva) and retrosternal discomfort.

A pharyngeal pouch is a posterior pharyngeal pulsion diverticulum through the Killian's dehiscence, usually seen in the 5-6th decade. The diagnosis is confirmed on Barium swallow. Treatment is endoscopic stapling of the pouch.

Plummer Vinson syndrome, also called Patterson Brown Kelly syndrome, consists of anaemia, glossitis, pharyngeal web, koilonychia and splenomegaly.

Post-cricoid tumours present with obstructive symptoms and loss of weight in the 5-6th decade. Laryngeal crepitus is lost in post-cricoid tumours and there may be widening of the laryngeal framework. The prognosis is not good.

Progressive bulbar palsy is more common in women causing dysphagia and dysarthria. The classical sign is fasciculation and wasting of the tongue. No treatment has any effect on the course of the disease.

Answer 6   A2, B1, C4, D3

The most common site of hypopharyngeal cancer is the pyriform fossa. These tumours usually present late and with a neck mass.

Lymphoma is usually seen in young adults with typical painless rubbery lymph nodes. The diagnosis is made by lymph node biopsy.

Glandular fever (infectious mononucelosis) is caused by Epstein Barr virus, and is a disease of young adults. The clinical features are sore throat, enlarged lymph nodes and hepatosplenomegaly.

Laryngocele forms as a result of an out-pouching from the laryngeal ventricle. It can be associated with carcinoma or papilloma of the larynx, which acts as a valve allowing air under pressure into the ventricle. The treatment is surgical excision.

Answer 7   A4, B1, C2, D3

Acute tonsillitis is a disease of children and young adults, commonly caused by ß haemolytic *Streptococcus*. The predominant symptom is sore throat that is made worse by swallowing. Penicillin is the most effective treatment for tonsillitis.

Tonsillar malignancy presents as a unilateral enlargement of a tonsil (which may be covered with slough) and an enlarged cervical lymph node in an elderly person. The common malignancy is squamous cell carcinoma.

Quinsy is another term for peritonsillar abscess. It follows an untreated acute tonsillitis, leading to pus collection lateral to the tonsil. Two or more attacks of quinsy are an indication for tonsillectomy. The treatment of quinsy is IV antibiotics and drainage of the abscess.

Gastroesophageal reflux disease can cause sore throat. The acid contents from the stomach regurgitate and irritate the pharynx and the larynx. The patient improves on treating the reflux.

Answer 8   A2, B1, C4, D3

Laryngeal cancer should always be ruled out in any elderly person presenting with a persistent hoarseness. The commonest malignancy is squamous cell carcinoma. The treatment is by radiotherapy or surgery depending on the staging of the tumour.

Vocal cord nodule is a benign condition seen in teachers and singers. It is seen at the junction of anterior 1/3 and posterior 2/3 of the vocal cord. It results from vocal abuse or misuse. Treatment is microlaryngeal surgery and speech therapy.

Reinke's oedema is the accumulation of fluid under the epithelium of true vocal cords. The cause is allergy, infections or cigarette smoking. Treatment is a combination of surgery and vocal rehabilitative measures.

Chronic sinusitis can cause hoarseness as the infected post-nasal discharge causes laryngitis leading to inflamed vocal cords.

Answer 9   A5, B4, C2, D3, E1

Submandibular duct stones are more common than parotid duct stones. This is so because the submandibular gland is a mixed seromucinous gland and is high in calcium, so epithelial debris calcifies easily.

Mumps is a viral infection of the parotid gland seen in young children. It is a very painful condition and the child is systemically quite unwell. Treatment is supportive.

Pleomorphic adenoma is the most common benign tumour of the salivary glands. It possesses epithelial and myoepithelial elements arranged in a mucopolysaccharide stroma. The treatment is surgical removal with a margin.

Adenoid cystic carcinoma is the most common malignant salivary neoplasm. It is more common in submandibular and sublingual glands. It characteristically spreads along the nerve sheaths. Management is the widest possible excision followed by radiotherapy.

Keratoconjunctivitis sicca syndrome or Sjogren's syndrome is a multisystem immunological condition affecting eyes, oral cavities and salivary glands. It is characterised by dry eyes, dry mouth and enlargement of salivary glands.

Answer 10   A5, B1, C4, D3, E2

Toxic nodular goitre presents with symptoms of hyperthyroidism and an enlarged thyroid gland in a young female. Management is primarily of the hyperthyroidism and then the nodule.

Endemic goitre is usually seen as a result of prolonged iodine deficiency causing hypothyroidism. The patient presents with the features of hypothyroidism and an enlarged thyroid gland.

Hashimoto's thyroiditis is an autoimmune disease of the thyroid characterised by anti thyroglobulin antibodies.

Thyroid malignancy should be ruled out in any patient with a rapidly growing thyroid gland. Papillary carcinoma is the most common thyroid malignancy followed by follicular, medullary and anaplastic. Anaplastic has the worst prognosis.

Medullary carcinoma is a tumour of parafollicular or C cells and is of neuroectodermal origin. It is characterised by elevation of serum calcitonin. Total thyroidectomy is the treatment of choice.

Answer 11   A4, B1, C2, D3

Acoustic neuroma should be ruled out in any adult with an asymmetrical sensorineural hearing loss. Acoustic neuroma is a tumour of the vestibular branch of the VIIIth cranial nerve in the internal auditory meatus (IAM). It is a slow-growing tumour and is diagnosed by MRI scan of the IAM. Treatment is by surgical excision.

Presbycusis is the term used for age-induced hearing loss seen in elderly people. Tinnitus is a common symptom associated with sensorineural hearing loss.

Ménière's disease, also known as endolymphatic hydrops is a disease of the inner ear. It is caused by excess production or inadequate absorption of endolymph. Treatment is both medical and surgical with an operation on the endolymphatic sac.

Glomus jugulare is a collection of ganglionic tissue in close relation to the jugular bulb within the temporal bone. It is diagnosed by CT and angiography. Treatment is surgical excision.

Answer 12   A2, B4, C1, D3

Benign positional paroxysmal vertigo is characterised by sudden onset of short-duration vertigo and nystagmus in a particular position of the head. It results because of displacement of some otoliths out of the ampulla of the semicircular canals. Treatment is with Epley's manoeuvre to replace otoliths into the ampulla.

Vertebrobasilar insufficiency can cause sudden onset of vertigo and drop attacks without loss of consciousness. It is usually associated with diabetes or atherosclerosis.

Vestibular neuronitis results because of viral infection of the vestibular ganglion located in the internal auditory canal. It manifests clinically by sudden onset of sustained vertigo lasting 3-7 days followed by gradual resolution. These vestibular signs occur in the absence of involvement of the auditory system.

Perilymph fistula means a fistula in the bony semicircular canal, resulting in exposure of the membranous semicircular canal. The characteristic symptom is change of hearing associated with feeling of fullness, tinnitus and disequilibrium. Treatment is to close the fistula at the earliest opportunity.

Answer 13   A2, B3, C4, D1

Bell's palsy is an idiopathic unilateral lower motor neurone facial palsy. It has an excellent prognosis with 90% patients recovering completely.

Ramsay Hunt syndrome is characterised by unilateral facial palsy and blisters on the pinna and ear canal. It is caused by the Herpes zoster virus. Treatment is with acyclovir.

Severe head injury can cause longitudinal or transverse fractures of the temporal bone. If the fracture line passes through the facial canal it can cause complete facial palsy.

Cholesteatoma is characterised by prolonged foul-smelling scanty ear discharge. Cholesteatoma can erode the bony facial canal and cause facial palsy. Treatment is mastoid exploration, removal of cholesteatoma and facial nerve decompression at the earliest opportunity.

Answer 14   A3, B1, C5, D4, E2

Otitis externa is dermatitis of the skin lining the ear canal and the pinna. It is usually a part of generalised eczema. It is usually bilateral and keeps flaring up off and on. The treatment is by keeping the affected skin dry and applying steroid antibiotic ointments.

Malignant otitis externa is a serious external and middle ear infection seen in diabetics. The causative organism is *Pseudomonas*. It can result in facial nerve palsy. It has to be treated aggressively.

Acute otitis media is a common childhood condition. The patient presents with a history of upper respiratory tract infection followed by a severe earache. The treatment is with antibiotics and decongestants. If not treated in time, the ear starts discharging and the pain is relieved.

Cholesteatoma is characterised by prolonged foul-smelling scanty ear discharge. It can be associated with a polyp arising from the middle ear. The treatment is mastoid exploration.

Acute mastoiditis is a complication of untreated acute or chronic otitis media. It manifests as pain and swelling behind the ear and the pinna is pushed outwards and forward. It has to be treated aggressively with IV antibiotics. If the patient does not respond to antibiotics in 48 hours, mastoid exploration has to be done.

Answer 15   A3, B4, C5, D1, E2

Impacted wax can cause earache due to a pressure effect as the skin of the ear canal is very sensitive. The self-cleansing mechanism of wax cleaning does not function in people using hearing aids as the aid acts as a mechanical obstruction.

Perichondritis is an infection of the perichondrium of the pinna and ear canal. It commonly occurs when the cartilage is exposed by trauma or surgery. It is a very painful condition as the perichondrium is tightly adherent to the underlying ear cartilage. It should be treated aggressively with antibiotics. If not treated promptly, it can result in necrosis of the ear cartilage causing ear deformity.

Bullous myringitis is a viral infection of the tympanic membrane. It manifests as purple blebs (haemorrhagic effusion) on the tympanic membrane and skin of the deep meatus. The patient presents with severe earache and serosanguinous discharge. Treatment is symptomatic.

The temporomandibular joint can be commonly involved in rheumatoid and osteoarthritis. The patient complains of earache as the auricular branch of the auriculotemporal nerve supplies both the TMJ and the pinna.

The eustachian tube equalises the pressure in the middle ear with the external atmosphere. Eustachian tube dysfunction can cause negative middle ear pressure. It manifests as earache and blockade sensation in the ear. It commonly follows upper respiratory tract infection and result in mucosal oedema of the nasal end of the eustachian tube. Treatment is by oral and topical decongestants.

Answer 16   A3, B5, C1, D2, E4

Myringoplasty is performed to patch up the tympanic membrane perforation. It can be performed by endaural or postaural route. Temporal fascia is usually used as the graft material for the operation. Success rates are in the range of 90%.

Cholesteatoma is treated by mastoidectomy. It involves clearing all the disease by complete removal of the cholesteatoma, diseased mastoid air cells and the involved ossicles. The primary aim of the operation is to make the ear safe and dry (hearing preservation is only secondary).

Menière's disease (endolymphatic hydrops) if not responding to medical treatment is treated by endolymphatic sac decompression. Decompression of the endolymphatic sac results in relief of vertigo and preservation of hearing.

Otosclerosis results in fixation of the stapes footplate in the oval window as a result of new bone formation. Stapedectomy involves removing the stapes and replacing it with a prosthesis that then conducts the sound to the inner ear.

Glue ear (otitis media with effusion) is treated with myringotomy (incision in the tympanic membrane) +/- grommet insertion. The fluid in the middle ear is sucked out and the grommet ventilates the middle ear.

Answer 17   A6, B5, C1, D2, E3, F4

Presbycusis is hearing loss in the elderly, of gradual onset and forms part of the progressive deterioration of the physiological function associated with the aging process. Tinnitus is caused by the hearing loss.

A nasopharyngeal tumour must be ruled out in any middle-aged person with conductive hearing loss with an intact ear drum. The tumour blocks the nasal end of the eustachian tube and causes effusion in the middle ear resulting in conductive hearing loss.

Glue ear (otitis media with effusion) is a very common cause of conductive hearing loss in children. It is a self-resolving process in children. Treatment is grommet insertion if bilateral glue persists for more than 4-6 months, so that the child's hearing is restored and speech development is not affected.

Otosclerosis affects young females. It causes fixation of the stapes footplate in the oval window causing immobility of the ossicular chain. It gives rise to deafness and vestibular symptoms. Characteristic finding on audiogram is a dip at 2000 Hz (Carhart's notch). Treatment is by a stapedectomy or a hearing aid.

Noise-induced hearing loss: repeated exposure to high levels of noise may cause sensory cell damage by direct mechanical action and by metabolic disturbances. The characteristic finding on audiogram is a dip at 4000 Hz frequency on the affected side.

Ototoxic drugs (Gentamycin) cause hearing loss by toxic degeneration of the inner hair cells. The initial manifestation is high frequency and continuous tinnitus followed by high frequency sensorineural hearing loss. The blood levels of amino glycosides must be carefully monitored and the dose adjusted to avoid damage to the inner ear.

Answer 18   A4, B5, C1, D2, E3

Allergic rhinitis is a IgE mediated hypersensitivity disease of the mucous membrane of the nasal airway characterised by sneezing, nasal blockade and discharge. Nasal blockade is because of bilateral inferior turbinate hypertrophy. Allergic rhinitis is mostly found in association with exposure to aeroallergens. Allergic rhinitis is either seasonal (summer hayfever) or perennial. Treatment is with oral antihistamines and topical nasal steroids.

Inverted papilloma is usually found unilaterally with male predominance commonly in the fifth decade. Appearance is of a reddish strawberry-like polyp arising from the lateral nasal wall. An important feature is their tendency to undergo malignant change (2-5% cases). Treatment is wide surgical excision and careful follow-up.

Choanal atresia is caused by failure of canalisation of the posterior choanae. Bilateral choanal atresia is a neonatal emergency as newborns are obligate nasal breathers. Unilateral choanal atresia can go unnoticed into adulthood. Treatment is surgical correction of the atresia.

Chronic sinusitis results in a foul-smelling nasal discharge, persistent post-nasal discharge and facial pains. Treatment is initially by antibiotics and decongestants. If no response is achieved, endoscopic sinus surgery is done to improve drainage and ventilation of the sinuses.

Nasal trauma can cause haematoma between the perichondrium and cartilage of the nasal septum leading to nasal obstruction. Treatment is drainage of the haematoma. If not drained, it can cause necrosis of the septal cartilage leading to a saddle deformity of the nose.

Answer 19   A4, B1, C2, D3

Sinonasal malignancy should always be ruled out in any elderly person presenting with nosebleeds. Cancer of nasal cavities or the paranasal sinuses is a highly lethal condition. Treatment is with radiotherapy and surgical resection.

Epistaxis may be the presenting feature of a patient on warfarin with a high international normalized ratio (INR). A high INR prevents blood clotting after a vessel starts bleeding from the nose. In addition to cauterising/packing the nose, warfarin dosage has to be adjusted to lower the INR.

Metastatic tumours in the nose/sinuses can present as epistaxis due to a friable nature of the tumour.

Hereditary haemorrhagic telangiectasia (Osler's disease) is a familial hereditary disease. It is recognised as red spots on the lips and mucous membranes of the mouth, tongue and telangiectasis on the face and in the nose. The defects in the nose are liable to cause severe epistaxis. Treatment is with carbon dioxide laser or by replacement of the septal mucous membrane by a split skin graft.

Answer 20   A3, B1, C4, D2

Chronic sinusitis results in a foul-smelling nasal discharge, persistent post-nasal discharge and facial pain. Treatment is initially by antibiotics and decongestants. If no response is achieved, endoscopic sinus surgery is done to improve drainage and ventilation of the sinuses.

Migraine is an important differential diagnosis of facial pain and headache. Pain may be accompanied by visual disturbances, motor and sensory symptoms, confusion and vomiting.

Trigeminal neuralgia is a paroxysmal sharp, needle-like pain on the face in the distribution of the trigeminal nerve. Any movement of the face may trigger a paroxysm. It may affect one or more divisions of the trigeminal nerve. Treatment is with Carbamezapine.

Post-herpetic neuralgia also occurs in the distribution of the trigeminal nerve after herpes zoster.

Answer 21   A3, B4, C1, D2

A nasal polyp results from the prolapsed lining of ethmoid sinuses and a blocked nose to variable degree. They appear as pale bags arising from the mucous membrane and are insensitive to touch. Treatment is a combination of surgery and medical therapy.

Allergic rhinitis is of two types: seasonal (summer hayfever) and perennial. It is characterised by watery nasal discharge, sneezing bouts and itching/irritation in the nose and eyes. Treatment is with antihistamines.

CSF rhinorrhoea manifests as clear watery fluid dripping through the nose after severe head injury. The fluid tests positive for glucose. The diagnostic test is its positivity for ß2 transferrin.

Poorly controlled diabetics are prone to getting chronic sinusitis with symptoms such as headache, postnasal discharge and rhinorrhoea.

Answer 22   A4, B1, C2, D3

Cystic fibrosis is a multisystem disorder. Nasal polyps arising before 10 years of age may be a presenting complaint of cystic fibrosis.

Sinonasal malignancy may present as a reddish, irregular polyp that bleeds on touching and is friable in an elderly person. Diagnosis is by biopsy of the lesion.

An antrochoanal polyp is a polyp that originates from the maxillary antrum and extends into the nasal cavity and towards the choanae. Treatment is by removal of the polyp. These polyps have a tendency for reccurence.

Endoscopic sinus surgery aims at improving the drainage and ventilation of sinuses. Recurrent nasal polyps should be treated with endoscopic ethmoidectomy for long-term benefit.

Chapter 15

Neurosurgery

Robert Redfern, FRCS

Consultant Neurosurgeon, Morriston Hospital, Swansea, UK

For all questions each option may be used once, more than once or not at all.

Question 1. Neuro-ophthamology

From each of the physical signs select the most likely cause from the options listed.

Options

1   Suprasellar extension of pituitary adenoma.
2   Pancoast tumour of (L) lung.
3   Left occipital lobe infarction.
4   Right occipital lobe infarction.
5   Right posterior temporal lobe tumour.
6   Right posterior communicating artery aneurysm.
7   Left posterior communicating artery aneurysm.
8   Myaesthenia gravis.

Stems

A   Left homonomous hemianopia.
B   Left superior quadrantanopia.
C   Bitemporal heminanopia.
D   Painful left third nerve palsy.
E   Left Horner's syndrome (meiosis, ptosis, decreased facial sweating).
F   Bilateral ptosis.

Question 2. Spinal syndromes

For each diagnosis give the most likely cause from the options listed.

Options

1   Slowly progressive reduction in walking distance with brisk lower limb reflexes and difficulty ascending stairs.
2   Acute onset of low back pain and unilateral foot drop.
3   Slowly progressive reduction in walking distance and absent lower limb reflexes.
4   Acute onset of low back pain with perineal numbness.
5   Severe dorsal pain with lower limb and trunk numbness.
6   Bilateral calf pain on walking 100 yards and relieved by rest.

Stems

A   Lumbar spinal stenosis.
B   Metastatic disease of spine.
C   Cervical myelopathy.
D   Posterolateral disc lesion.
E   Central lumbar disc herniation.
F   Intermittent claudication.

Question 3. Upper limb pain syndromes

For each symptom/sign listed choose the most likely diagnosis from the options listed.

Options

1   (R) parietal metastatic tumour.
2   (L) C5/6 disc lesion.
3   (L) ulnar nerve lesion at elbow.
4   (L) carpal tunnel syndrome.
5   Syringomyelia.
6   Reflex sympathetic dystrophy (regional pain syndrome).

Stems

A   Dissociated sensory loss with hand and arm weakness.
B   Painful nocturnal numbness of (L) thumb, index and middle fingers.
C   Weak (L) biceps muscle.
D   Pain and numbness of (L) little and ring fingers.
E   Painful stiff hand with warm, mottled skin.

Question 4. Acute neurological syndromes

For each clinical scenario give the most likely cause from the listed options.

Options

1   Sudden onset of severe headache and neck stiffness.
2   Sudden onset of right hemiparesis and aphasia, without headache.
3   Rapid development of unilateral headache, nausea and visual disturbance.
4   Gradual onset of hemiparesis and personality change.
5   Sudden onset of painless paraparesis and urinary retention.

Stems

A   Classical migraine.
B   Spinal cord infarction.
C   Ischaemic stroke.
D   Aneurysmal subarachnoid haemorrhage.
E   Frontal neoplasm.

Question 5. Neurocutaneous syndromes

Match the diagnosis with the syndromes from the listed options.

Options

1   Epilepsy, mental retardation and sebaceous adenoma.
2   Multiple cutaneous nodules and bilateral acoustic neuromas.
3   Port wine facial stain and cerebral arteriovenous malformation.
4   Cerebellar cystic tumour with mural nodule and renal adenocarcinoma.

Stems

A   von Hippel Lindau syndrome.
B   Neurofibromatosis Type II.
C   Sturge-Weber syndrome.
D   Tuberous sclerosis.

Question 6. Intracranial infection

From the list of infective conditions of the central nervous system choose the most likely cause from the options listed. Each answer should be used once only.

Options

1   Dental sepsis.
2   Bronchiectasis.
3   Mastoidectomy.
4   Neonatal infection.
5   Pulmonary tuberculosis.

Stems

A   Temporal lobe abscess.
B   Aseptic meningitis.
C   Occipital lobe abscess.
D   Subdural empyema.
E   Cavernous sinus thrombosis.

Question 7. CSF analysis

From the list of options select the most likely diagnosis from the CSF analysis below.

Options

1   Tuberculous meningitis.
2   Viral meningitis.
3   Bacterial meningitis.
4   Carcinomatous meningitis.

Stems

A   6 lymphocytes; glucose 0.6; protein 0.2.
B   180 polymorphs; glucose 0.3; protein 0.6
C   80 lymphocytes and 40 polymorphs; glucose 0.2; protein 2.0.
D   Atypical cells; glucose 0.25; protein 0.8.

(Normal ranges: <5 WBCs per mm^3; glucose $0\cdot45 - 0\cdot7$ g/L; protein $0\cdot15$-$0\cdot45$ g/L).

Question 8. Ocular signs with altered consciousness

For each group of signs choose the most likely diagnosis from the options listed. Each answer should be used once only.

Options

1   Extradural haematoma.
2   Subarachnoid haemorrhage.
3   Pontine haemorrhage.
4   Non-specific raised intracranial pressure (eg. hemisphere tumour or hydrocephalus).

Stems

A   Pinpoint unreactive pupils and coma.
B   Widely dilated unreactive pupil with contralateral hemiparesis and drowsiness.
C   Normally reacting pupils, retinal haemorrhages and drowsiness.
D   Normally reacting pupils, unilateral lateral rectus palsy, and drowsiness.

Question 9. Neuroradiology

For each of the radiological appearances select the most likely diagnostic option from those listed below. Each answer should be used once only.

Options

1   Colloid cyst.
2   Haemangioblastoma.
3   Meningioma.
4   Chromophobe adenoma.
5   Glioblastoma multiforme.
6   Schwannoma.
7   Medulloblastoma.

Stems

A   Smooth enhancing lesion of the sphenoid wing.
B   Small enhancing lesion of the anterior IIIrd ventricle with associated obstructive hydrocephalus.
C   Enhancing lesion within the pituitary fossa.
D   Midline lesion of the cerebellum in a child with obstructive hydrocephalus.
E   Enhancing nodule within the wall of a cystic lesion of the cerebellum in an adult.
F   Enhancing lesion, partly cystic, of the cerebello-pontine angle.
G   Irregular enhancing lesion of the anterior corpus callosum.

Question 10. Dementia

From the list of options select the most likely diagnosis from the causes of dementia listed below. Each option should be used once only.

Options

1   Normal pressure hydrocephalus.
2   Alzheimer's disease.
3   Multiple infarct dementia.
4   Frontal lobe tumour.
5   Carotid stenosis.

Stems

A   A progressive story of dementia, gait disturbance, and urinary incontinence with CT evidence of generalised ventricular enlargment (hydrocephalus) with relative sparing of the cortical sulci.
B   A progressive story of confusion, lower limb weakness and altered sense of smell.
C   Progressive dementia with CT evidence of generalised ventricular enlargment and wide cortical sulci.
D   Progressive dementia with CT evidence of generalised ventricular enlargement with scattered low density areas in the cortex.
E   Transient ischaemic attacks.

Question 11. Movement disorders

From the options listed select the most likely diagnosis from those listed below. Each diagnosis should be used once only.

Options

1   Parkinsonism.
2   Hemiballismus.
3   Chorea.
4   Athetosis.
5   Drug-induced dystonia.

Stems

A   Sustained abnormal posture of the head and neck, with upward deviation of the eyes.
B   Slow writhing movements of the limbs.
C   Slow jerking movements of the limbs.
D   Sudden violent movements of the limbs.
E   Coarse tremor of the upper limbs with rigidity, and paucity of facial expression.

Question 12. Neurological signs in lower limbs

From the options listed select the most likely nerve root responsible for the sign or symptom listed below.

Options

1   L3 nerve root.
2   L4 nerve root.
3   L5 nerve root.
4   S1 nerve root.
5   S2 nerve root.

Stems

A   Absent ankle jerk.
B   Absent knee jerk.
C   Numbness of great toe.
D   Numbness of outer border of foot.
E   Weakness of extension of great toe.
F   Weakness of knee flexion.

Question 13. Neurological signs in upper limbs

From the options listed select the most likely nerve root responsible for the sign or symptom listed below.

Options

1   C3 nerve root.
2   C4 nerve root.
3   C5 nerve root.
4   C6 nerve root.
5   C7 nerve root.
6   C8 nerve root.
7   T1 nerve root.

Stems

A   Triceps jerk.
B   Hoffman reflex and paraesthesia in ring and little fingers.
C   Numbness over dorsum of thumb.
D   Weakness of finger extrusion.
E   Weakness of finger abduction.

Question 14. Physical signs in neurosurgery

From the following list of physical signs select all those which may result from the diagnoses listed below. More than one answer may be selected for some of the diagnoses.

Options

1   CSF otorrhoea.
2   CSF rhinorrhoea.
3   Loss of sense of smell on clinical testing.
4   Battle's sign (retromastoid bruising).
5   Neck pain on active or passive flexion.
6   Neck stiffness due to subarachnoid blood.

Stems

A   Anterior fossa fracture due to a blow to the forehead from a large object suspended from an overhead gantry.

B   Fracture of petrous bone due to a direct blow to the temporal region.

C   Occipital fracture due to falling over backwards onto pavement whilst drunk.

D   Meningioma of olfactory groove.

E   Hydrocephalus due to congenital aqueduct stenosis.

Question 15. Spinal radiology

For each radiological sign choose the most likely diagnosis or diagnoses from the options listed below. Some signs may have more than one diagnosis and these should be selected where appropriate.

Options

1   Osteoporosis.
2   Spinal discitis.
3   Metastatic disease of vertebral body.
4   Spinal cord tumour.
5   Delayed effects of spinal trauma.
6   Lumbar stenosis.
7   None of the above.

Stems

A   Loss of disc space and kyphosis of mid-dorsal spine.
B   Paraspinal mass with acute vertebral body collapse.
C   Syringomyelia.
D   Vertebral collapse with preservation of disc space.
E   Spina bifida occulta.

Answer 1   A4, B5, C1, D7, E2, F8

Fibres from the nasal retina decussate in the optic chiasm to reach the contralateral geniculate body and, via the optic radiation, the contralateral occipital cortex. Some of the inferior fibres of the optic radiation (derived from the contralateral inferior nasal retina - and thus conveying information from the superior temporal field of vision, and from the ipsilateral inferior temporal retina, subserving the superior nasal field of vision) pass forwards in the posterior temporal region as Meyer's loop. In this position they may be vulnerable to damage from temporal lobe tumours, or surgery in this region.

Answer 2   A3, B5, C1, D2, E4, F6

NB. Cervical myelopathy causes spasticity with pyramidal weakness (proximal weakness in legs).

Central disc rupture at L4/5 can result in cauda equina syndrome which can cause sphincter disturbance, 'saddle anaesthesia' (sensory deficit over buttock and perineal region), motor weakness, bilateral absent ankle jerks and disturbance of sexual function.

Intermittent claudication is due to vascular insufficiency with pain occurring on walking and relieved by rest, an important factor to differentiate it from neurogenic claudication seen most commonly in lumbar canal stenosis.

Answer 3   A5, B4, C2, D3, E6.

Syringomyelia is cystic cavitation of the spinal cord. It may be associated with certain congenital or neoplastic conditions or may follow significant spinal trauma with or without spinal cord injury. Characteristic syndromes include sensory loss, cervical or occipital pain, lower motor neurone hand and arm weakness, and painless arthropathies.

Answer 4   A3, B5, C2, D1, E4.

Note that there is significant diagnostic overlap so that urgent investigation of most such cases should be arranged. Note also that there is no such condition as a 'sentinel subarachnoid haemorrhage' (in much the same way as there is no such thing as a 'sentinel pregnancy'!).

Answer 5   A4, B2, C3, D1

Neurofibromatosis Type II should be distinguished from Type I (also known as von Recklinghausen disease). Hallmarks of Type I are café-au-lait spots, hyper-pigmentation, optic glioma, Lisch nodules. Bilateral acoustic nerve tumours are virtually non-existent in Type I, but diagnostic of Type II.

In tuberous sclerosis, intracranial calcification is seen in the sub-ependymal region as a nodule (tuber) or hamartoma.

Answer 6   A3, B5, C2, D4, E1

Venous drainage from the mouth and face includes communication into the cavernous sinus. Bronchiectasis may result in haematogenous spread of organisms to the brain and, in the absence of a local cause, occipital lobe abscesses are usually the result of such spread. Mastoidectomy may result in direct dural damage or transmission of infection may be via infective venous spread.

Answer 7   A2, B3, C1, D4

Answer 8   A3, B1, C2, D4

Isolated sixth nerve palsy is a false localising sign of raised intracranial pressure. It can also result from cavernous sinus lesions, vasculopathy etc. Non-pupil-sparing third nerve palsy can result from tumours, aneurysms, uncal herniation or cavernous sinus problems.

Answer 9   A3, B1, C4, D7, E2, F6, G5

Note that although meningiomas and gliomas can occur at many sites they, like other tumours, are more commonly found at specific sites. Some tumours, eg. acoustic Schwannoma (neuroma) and pituitary adenomas, are clearly found at specific sites. Medulloblastomas are characteristically located in the posterior fossa in the midline in childhood, but more laterally, within the cerebellar hemispheres, in adults. Haemangioblastoma usually presents as a cystic cerebellar hemisphere lesion with an enhancing (vascular) mural nodule, but it may be encountered within the cerebral hemispheres or spinal cord or within the vermis.

Answer 10   A1, B4, C2, D3, E5

Only 10-20% of all cases of dementia are caused by a treatable condition. Intoxication, infection, vascular and metabolic abnormalities can contribute. Alzheimer's disease (also known as senile dementia) causes atrophy of cerebral convolutions resulting in aphasia, apraxia, agnosia and dementia.

Answer 11   A5, B4, C3, D2, E1

Answer 12   A4, B2, C3, D4, E3, F4

It is important to remember that in the lumbar region the nerve root exits below and in close proximity to the pedicle of the like number vertebra. A herniated lumbar disc usually spares the nerve root exiting at that interspace and impinges on the nerve exiting from the neural foramen one level below i.e. L5/S1 disc usually causes S1 radiculopathy.

Answer 13   A5, B6, C4, D5, E7

Answer 14   A2, 3, 5 & 6, B1, 2, 4, 5 & 6, C5 & 6, D2 & 3, E2

Most basal skull fractures are extensions of fractures through the cranial vault. Signs include CSF otorrhoea or rhinorrhoea, haemotympanum, post-auricular ecchymosis (Battle's sign), periorbital ecchymoses (raccoon's eyes) and cranial nerve involvement.

Answer 15   A2 & 3, B2 & 3, C4 & 5, D1 & 3, E7

Patients with discitis have severe back pain exacerbated by movement, fever and paravertebral spasms and elevated ESR, CRP and WBC.

Spinal metastases occur in 10% of all cancer patients. 80% of primary sites are lungs, breast, GI, prostate, melanoma and lymphoma.

Chapter 16
Transplantation surgery

Gareth Tervit, FRCS
Consultant Vascular Surgeon
University Hospital of North Durham, Durham, UK

For all questions each option may be used once, more than once or not at all.

Question 1. Brain stem death

Options

1 Unconsciousness.
2 Asystole.
3 Spontaneous respiration.
4 Hypothermia.
5 Hypernatraemia.

Stems

A Presence of this is essential for the diagnosis of brain stem death (BSD).
B May be present but inadequate in BSD.
C This follows soon after BSD.
D A diagnosis of death may not be made if this is present.
E Is defined as a Glasgow coma scale of less than 8.

Question 2. Brain stem death

Options

1   V.
2   VII.
3   VIII.
4   II.
5   III.

Stems

A   This afferent nerve is tested with a bright light.
B   This efferent nerve is tested with corneal stimulation.
C   This afferent nerve is stimulated with instillation of ice cold water.
D   This efferent nerve is tested with a bright light.
E   Stimulation of this nerve's somatic area should not evoke a response.

Question 3. Brain stem death

Options

1   Loss of knee/ankle jerks.
2   Restoration of normothermia.
3   Allowing time for drug metabolism.
4   Testing respiratory effort by raising the PCO_2 to 5 Kpa in the absence of ventilation.
5   Electroencephalography showing no activity.

Stems

A   A 20-year-old male overdoses on diazepam, amitryptiline and paracetamol, and is found by police to be hypothermic in a doorway. He is resuscitated with mouth-to-mouth prior to ventilation and transport to ITU. There is no response 24 hours later to maintenance therapy. The question of brain death is raised. What is necessary before this can be diagnosed?
B   Which criteria are not part of the diagnosis of brain stem death?

Question 4. Organ transplantation

Options

1   Are relative contraindications to tissue donation.
2   Are total contraindications to tissue donation.
3   Requires special preparation and management prior to harvesting.
4   Can be used if the recipient is compatible.
5   Increases the risk of malignancy.

Stems

A   Hep B or hep C positive donors.
B   HIV or systemic sepsis.
C   Refusal of consent.
D   Non-heart beating donor.
E   CMV infection in the donor.

Question 5. Transplant nephrectomy

Options

1   Pain.
2   Haematuria.
3   Infection.
4   Sensitisation.
5   Hyperacute rejection.

Stems

A   Which indications would suggest an approach to remove all foreign tissue?
B   Which indications would probably necessitate a subcapsular approach?
C   What is the indication which should improve the survival of further transplants?

Question 6. Grafts

Options

1   A graft originating from and applied to the same individual.
2   A graft between two animals of different species.
3   A graft between two genetically identical individuals.
4   A graft between two genetically dissimilar individuals of the same species.

Stems

A   An allograft is ...
B   A syngenic graft is ...
C   A xenograft is ...
D   An autograft is ...
E   An isograft is ...

Question 7. Immunology

Options

1   The ABO antigens.
2   The major histocompatibility complex.
3   Human leucocyte antigens.

Stems

A   These are found in the MHC part of the human genome.
B   Their principal function is to display peptide antigens for recognition by T cells.
C   All mammals have these.
D   These are found on glycolipids expressed on the surface of erythrocytes.
E   There are three classes of these.

Question 8. Blood group compatibility

Options

1   A.
2   B.
3   O.
4   AB.
5   AO.

Stems

A   Universal blood donor.
B   Universal recipient.
C   A patient with this blood group could not receive type B blood.

Question 9. The donor

Options

1   Would be suitable for a renal transplant.
2   Would not be suitable for renal transplantation.
3   Would need further specialist work-up before being considered.

Stems

A   A 20-year-old woman with AIDS.
B   An 80-year-old man with end-stage hypertensive renal failure.
C   A 65-year-old woman with Dukes B rectal cancer at age 55.
D   A 57-year-old male with advanced dialysis accelerated atherosclerosis.
E   A 26-year-old illegal immigrant with pulmonary TB which is drug-sensitive.

Question 10. Organ preservation in renal transplant donors

Options

1 Universally aids organ preservation.
2 Produces prompt and difficult to resuscitate cardiac arrest.
3 Is not used as a preservative.
4 Was developed at the University of Wales.
5 Stimulates the production of Desmopressin (DDAVP).

Stems

A Intra-arterial UW solution.
B Intravenous Hartmann's solution.
C Intra-arterial Collins solution.
D Intravenous Collins solution.
E None of the above.

Question 11. Organ preservation

Options

1 Cell swelling.
2 Facilitation of the sodium potassium pump.
3 Membrane stability.
4 Thickening of cellular membranes.
5 Thinning of mitochondrial membranes.

Stems

A Hypothermic preservation causes ...
B Deficiency of adenosine tri-phosphate is responsible for ...
C Use of an osmotic agent in the preservation solution causes ...

Question 12. Organ preservation

In a warm ischaemic kidney.

Options

1   18 hours.
2   30 minutes.
3   72 hours.
4   2 hours.
5   None of the above.

Stems

A   The available time before deterioration in renal function is ...
B   Depletion of ADP causes tissue damage in ...
C   If properly preserved the kidney can be used up to ...
D   Na-K ATPase initiates cell swelling within ...
E   H-K ATPase initiates cellular swelling in ...

Question 13. Preservative solutions

In order to try to preserve cell function the following are used in solution.

Options

1   Maintains intracellular potassium.
2   Keeps cellular swelling to a minimum.
3   Allows a good supply of ATP on reperfusion.
4   Buffers the products of anaerobic metabolism.

Stems

A   A potassium concentration of 120mmol.
B   Adenosine.
C   Phosphate.
D   Hyper-tonic glucose or starch polymer.

Question 14. Cellular rejection

Options

1   B cell receptor complex.
2   T cell receptor complex.
3   Intracytoplasmic enzyme.
4   Surface glycoproteins on T cells.
5   CD3 complex and in combination with this forms a unit capable of intracytoplasmic signalling.

Stems

A   CD4 and CD8 are ...
B   HLA binds to ...
C   Alloantigen is presented to ...
D   TCR is associated with ...
E   ZAP-70 is a type of ...

Question 15. Immunology

There are two allorecognition pathways.

Options

1   The direct allorecognition pathway.
2   The parallel allorecognition pathway.
3   The indirect allorecognition pathway.
4   The Krebs pathway.

Stems

A   The donor Antigen Presenting Cell and HLA is involved in ...
B   The recipient APC and donor allopeptide is involved in ...
C   Recipient T cells are involved with ...
D   A normal immune response progression is similar to ...

Question 16. Rejection

Options

1   Duplex scan.
2   Biopsy.
3   Bladder scan/washout.
4   Temperature, pulse and blood pressure.
5   Cyclosporin levels.

Stems

A   2 hours after surgery to implant an allogenic kidney the urine output is found to tail off. The surgeon is called and he orders some investigations. Which ones would you perform?

B   The other kidney recipient from this donor does well until 6 weeks post-transplant when her renal function deteriorates. Which tests would be more useful now?

Question 17. Rejection

Options

1   Occurs within hours.
2   Occurs within days or weeks.
3   Occurs after 6 months.
4   May be due to ABO incompatibility.
5   Is due to CD8 deficiency.

Stems

A   Chronic rejection.
B   Hyper-acute rejection.
C   Acute rejection.
D   Cell mediated immunity causes a rejection which typically ...

Question 18. Rejection

The graft blood vessels are the site of change in all types of rejection. Which changes are typical of which type of rejection process?

Options

1   Complement activation and activation of the endothelium.
2   Margination, and migration of T cells, B cells, macrophages and NK cells.
3   Progressive myointimal proliferation.
4   Migration of the myointima into the loop of Henle.
5   Increasing fibrosis and ischaemia.
6   Intravascular thrombosis.

Stems

A   Acute rejection.
B   Chronic rejection.
C   Hyperacute rejection.

Question 19. Immunosuppression

Match the following immunosuppressants with their properties.

Options

1   Cyclosporin.
2   FK506.
3   Azathioprine.
4   OKT3.
5   Mycophenolate mofetil.

Stems

A   A 6 mercaptopurine analogue.
B   A calcineurin antagonist.
C   A murine antibody.
D   An antiproliferative agent

Question 20. Anti-rejection drugs

Match these to the appropriate drugs.

Options

1   Inhibition of T lymphocyte activation.
2   Inhibition of T and B cell proliferation.
3   Nephrotoxicity.
4   Requires drug monitoring.
5   All of the above.

Stems

A   Calcineurin antagonists.
B   Corticosteroids.
C   Azathioprine.
D   MMF.

Question 21. Drug regimes

Which drugs would you expect to give for immunosuppression in the following cases?

Options

1   Cyclosporin.
2   Prednisolone.
3   Azathioprine.
4   MMF.
5   OKT3.

Stems

A   A 47-year-old male receiving his first transplant for diabetes.
B   A 30-year-old mother of two receiving her second transplant.

Question 22. Liver transplantation

Options

1   A whole liver from a fit 35-year-old male who died from cerebral haemorrhage but was HIV positive (i.e. did not have AIDS).
2   The left lobe of liver from a living related donor.
3   A whole liver from a diabetic who had fatty infiltration (30%).
4   A half liver and kidney from a fit and healthy patient.
5   This patient is not suitable for transplantation.

Stems

A   A 2-year-old boy with biliary atresia whose Kasai procedeure is reaching the end of its useful function.
B   A 40-year-old woman with primary biliary cirrhosis and hepato-renal syndrome leading to renal failure.
C   A 35-year-old man with sclerosing cholangitis who needs complete liver resection to remove his cholangiocarcinoma.
D   A 60-year-old alcoholic with diabetic renal failure who has abstained for 12 months and otherwise is fit and well.

Question 23. Liver transplantation

You are called on to help harvest a donor. The transplant surgeon feels warm and steps outside for a breath of fresh air, telling you to carry on. The abdomen is opened and the ligaments of the liver are divided. You are dissecting the structures in the lesser omentum.

Options

1   The hepatic artery arises from the coeliac axis.
2   The right hepatic artery arises from the SMA.
3   The right hepatic artery arises from the left gastric artery.
4   The portal vein arises from the confluence of the IMV and the IVC.
5   The portal vein arises from the SMV and splenic vein.
6   The portal vein is the first structure found in the edge of the lesser omentum.

Stems

A   Which is the most likely situation to be found?
B   Which scenarios are the most unlikely?
C   Which are well-recognised anatomical variation(s)?

Question 24. Liver transplantation - acute complications

Options

1   Renal failure.
2   Poor bile production.
3   Acidosis.
4   Coagulopathy.
5   Bleeding.

Stems

A   Is/are common complication(s) due to clamping the IVC.
B   Is/are common signs in primary graft dysfunction - an emergency.
C   May be more common after transplanting for cirrhosis.
D   May herald thrombosis of the hepatic artery.

Question 25. Liver transplantation - infections

Options

1   Cytomegalovirus (CMV).
2   Nosocomial bacteria.
3   Candida.
4   *Pneumocystis carnii.*
5   Hepatitis B.

Stems

A   Common infective agent(s) in the first week.
B   Can be avoided by appropriate donor/recipient matching.
C   Can be usefully treated with gancyclovir.
D   Requires treatment with sulphamethoxazole and trimethoprim.
E   Treatment with immunoglobulin gives good results.

Question 26. Liver anatomy

Segmental and living donor transplantation is possible because of our knowledge of liver anatomy.

Options

1   The right hepatic vein.
2   The left hepatic vein.
3   The middle hepatic vein.
4   The falciform ligament.
5   The caudate lobe.
6   The quadrate lobe.
7   None of the above.

Stems

A   The liver is divided into functional right and left lobes by ..
B   The segment 1 of the caudate lobe is supplied by these veins.
C   The main branches of the portal vein are ...
D   Segments II and III are supplied by ...

Question 27. Transplanted organs

Transplanted organs are implanted into various sites. Fill in the blanks.

Options

1 Orthotopic.
2 Heterotopic.
3 Orthopaedic.
4 Extraperitoneal.

Stems

A Pancreases are transplanted into a XXXX site.
B This means transplantation into an abnormal site.
C Kidneys are transplanted into a XXXX site.
D Livers are typically described as XXXX transplants.

Question 28. Renal operative options

You have a left-sided donor kidney with a small accessory renal artery and a duplex ureter. Your registrar has several 'helpful suggestions'. Which should you ignore?

1 Tie off the accessory artery and implant in the left side of the recipient.
2 Discard the kidney as it is not usable.
3 Implant it in the right side of the donor.
4 Anastomose the ureters together before implantation.
5 Implant it in the left side of the donor.
6 Tie off the abnormal ureter.
7 Implant both ureters separately.
8 Anastomose the accessory artery to the renal artery and implant as usual.
9 Use the inferior epigastric artery to anastomose to the accessory artery.

Question 29. Living renal donors

Options

1   Cadaveric.
2   Living related.
3   Living unrelated.
4   HLA identical.
5   1 haplotype mismatch.

Stems

A   Which category tends to give the best result?
B   Which category would a younger brother possibly fit?
C   Which would give a patient the best chance of graft survival - a cadaveric graft or a graft from her husband?
D   Which category(s) would my monozygotic twin sister fit into?

Question 30. Ethics

Options

1   Yes.
2   No.

Stems

A   A 30-year-old has suffered an extensive intra-cranial bleed with loss of all brain stem reflexes. His respiration is becoming erratic and will shortly cease. With regards to our legal and ethical position should he be ventilated? He carries a donor card signed 5 years ago.

B   A 68-year-old male from a far eastern country has renal failure and no prospect of dialysis in his own country for various logistical reasons. He is rich and wishes to pay a donor for a kidney as none of his family are a suitable match. He approaches you as a surgeon. Should you act as his transplant surgeon?

References and further reading

1. Majid A, Kingsnorth A. *Advanced surgical practice*. GMM press, London, 2002.
2. Forsythe JLR. *Transplantation Surgery: Current Dilemmas*, 2nd edition. WB Saunders, London, 2001.

Answer 1   A1, B3, C2, D4, E1

Answer 2   A4, B2, C3, D5, E1

Answer 3   A2 & 3, B1, 4 & 5

Spinal reflexes may be preserved in brain stem death and EEG is not currently part of the criteria issued by the royal colleges. Raising the $paCO_2$ above 6.65 kpa is though. Drug metabolism may be significantly slowed by hypothermia, and liver damage and competitive metabolism in the liver.

Answer 4   A1 & 3, B2, C2, D3 & 4, E1, 4 & 5

Answer 5   A5, B1, 2, 3 & 4, C4

Kidneys rejected in 90 days tend to have the whole transplant removed. After this there are too many adhesions to easily and safely do this, so an extraperitoneal subcapsular approach is made instead. Grafts may be removed to prevent ongoing immune stimulation and generation of new antibodies which may prejudice further grafts.

Answer 6   A4, B3, C2, D1, E3

Answer 7   A3, B3, C2, D1, E3

Answer 8   A3, B4, C1, 3 & 5

Answer 9   A2, B2, C1, D3, E2

A, B, and E are all considered unsuitable for renal transplantation due to age and active infection. Patient C could be considered cured of her cancer and is suitable. Patient D would require further assessment of his iliac arteries.

Answer 10   A1, B3, C1, D2, E4

Answer 11   A1 & 3, B1 & 4, C3

Answer 12   A2, B5, C1, D2, E5

Upon the onset of ischaemia the cell quickly uses up its supply of ATP and this leads to failure of the Na-K ATPase and cellular swelling and water.

Answer 13   A1 & 2, B3, C3 & 4, D2

Answer 14   A4, B2, C2, D5, E3

Alloantigen is presented on the HLA molecule to the TCR complex. This in turn activates ZAP-70 which intitiates an intracytoplasmic response.

Answer 15   A1, B2, C1 & 2, D2

Answer 16   A1, 3 & 4, B2 & 5

Answer 17   A3, B1 & 4, C2, D2

Answer 18   A1, B3 & 5, C1 & 6

Answer 19   A3, B1 & 2, C4, D3 & 5

Answer 20   A1, 3 & 4, B1, C2, D2

Answer 21   A1, 2 & 3, B1, 2, 3, or 4 & 5

Initially patients are started on triple therapy (calcineurin antagonist, antiproliferative and steroid) and this is reduced as possible over time. The woman in B would probably be sensitised due to either her pregnancies or previous transplant and would require anti-lymphocyte globulin initially.

Answer 22   A2, B2 & 3, C5, D4

A   Living related transplant is increasing in frequency and is effective. The main concern is the safety of the donor.

B   In this situation a mildly diseased donor liver could be considered and the patient's kidneys would reasonably be expected to recover.

C   Survival in this situation is very poor and the patient should probably have been transplanted before his malignancy developed.

D   Dual organ transplantation is well-recognised and some surgeons would consider a pancreatic transplant at the same time to improve diabetic control.

HIV positive donors are not suitable although HIV positive patients (but not AIDS patients) are considered.

Answer 23   A1 & 5, B3, 4 & 6, C2

Hepatic arterial anatomy is variable with 70% of hepatic arteries arising from the coeliac axis. Common variations are a right hepatic arising from the SMA and a left hepatic from the left gastric. The hepatic artery may also arise from the SMA.

Answer 24   A1, B2, 3 & 4, C5, D2 & 4

Answer 25   A2, B1, C1, D4, E5

A   As with most operations bacterial infection is common in the first week and tends to be in the chest or biliary.

B,C CMV typing should ensure that infection from donor to recipient does not occur, but it can be treated with gancyclovir and immunosuppression reduction.

D   These are the component parts of septrin (co-trimoxazole), an anti-pneumocystis antibiotic.

E   In combination with the antiviral lamivudine, this is used to treat resurgence of hepatitis B.

Answer 26   A3, B1 & 2, C7, D2

Answer 27   A2 & 4, B2, C2 & 4, D1

Orthoptic transplants go into the same space as the original organs. Typically, the kidneys and pancreas are transplanted into the retro-peritoneal space.

Answer 28   1, 2, 4, 6

A donor kidney may be implanted in either side of a recipient but extension grafts may be necessary. The accessory renal artery is essential to the segment of the kidney it supplies and flow must be restored. Hopefully, the harvesting surgeon will have taken it as part of the Carrell patch but if not, then bench work or using other arteries are both options. Both ureters must be implanted but anastomosing them is a bad idea due to the poor blood supply and likelihood of leakage.

Answer 29   A4, B2 & 5, C3, D2 & 4

Living related donation is justifiable by the superiority of graft survival to cadaveric transplantation.

Answer 30   A2, B2

A   No. As he is still breathing he cannot undergo formal brain stem death testing and is not technically dead. If he is still alive then he cannot consent to what is a considerable upgrading in his treatment and if there is no hope of recovery then it cannot be said to be in his best interests. We cannot intervene on his behalf as healthcare professionals.

B   No. In the UK at the moment it is considered unethical and illegal to act as a surgeon when the donor gives an organ unless it is donated altruistically. It is felt that if this was encouraged then there would be a great tendency for the poorer classes and the 3rd world to be seen as an organ pool for richer classes and countries.